THE GREAT MEDICAL STUDENT Odyssey

TALES & ADVENTURES IN MEDICAL SCHOOL

ASHIQ PRAMCHAND

First published by Ashiq Pramchand, 2021

Copyright © 2021 by Ashiq Pramchand

978-0-620-91762-9 (e-book)
9780-620-91761-2 (print)

Cover Design and Typesetting by Gregg Davies Media
(www.greggdavies.com)

Additional copies of this book can be purchased
from all leading book retailers worldwide.

CONTENTS

1

HOW IT ALL STARTED

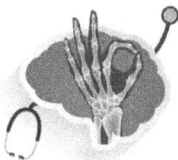

"The shortest answer is doing the thing."

— *ERNEST HEMINGWAY*

Would you believe me if I told you that I chased a chicken out of a hospital emergency room? Or that I spend most of my time covered in other people's blood? Or that my hospital team members fended off a psychiatric patient who threatened to stab all of us? I wouldn't blame you for thinking: "This guy is crazy for going through all this." I'll let you in on a little secret. These experiences are tame in comparison to some things that other medical students have seen...

Hi there! My name is Ashiq Pramchand. You might wonder: "Why am I sharing my personal medical school experiences with you?" When I arrived at the Nelson R. Mandela School of Medicine as a first-year student; I realized that I had no idea about what lay in store for me. I attended a private high school in KwaZulu natal, Durban (which is worlds apart from many of

South Africa's poorest rural schools). The last thing I wish to have is an ivory tower perspective of challenges that students experience daily. I hope that my medical school adventures can shed some light on our lives as medical students and inspire others to fall in love with medicine. I'm just one of many medical students who have amazing stories to tell.

When I first started writing this book, I was in my second year of medical school. In university, time seems to work in strange ways. It is easy to fall into a routine. Time feels accelerated. But everything seems to slow down when you only have 5 weeks to study everything about an organ system for a test…no pressure. Whenever I get some downtime, I like to write down my thoughts and capture the fleeting moments that make medical school such a memorable adventure. These writing sessions offer me a valuable opportunity to reflect on some of my more salient…and hilarious experiences.

But how was I thrust into this rollercoaster ride of a degree?

Even since my childhood, learning new things has fascinated me. I am not sure if this trait was innate or if my dad instilled it in me. Regardless, I strongly believe that this is a quality that can be developed over time. Sophocles said, "Always desire to learn something useful."

Primary school (grades 1-7) is somewhat of a blur for me. It was a socially awkward time for many of us. I realize now that it was a crucial period in which many of my habits for studying and making friends were forming. I cannot help but feel that it is easier to learn good habits when one is young. But it is never too late to change. It is easier to forge a sword when it is in a malleable state. Thereafter it may be sharpened.

In a way, I saw primary school as my, "malleable state." The competition was tough in our school. A ranking system for top students was clear. The students who worked the hardest and the smartest were rewarded for their endeavors in front of the entire school, with praise, medals, and trophies. My dad told me about the benefits of academic success. The general idea behind their advice was: if you perform well in school, you will improve your chances of being accepted at a prestigious university, which will improve your chances of finding a great job, which will lead to an overall successful life and so on and so forth. Many Indian families will say this. It is, of course, harder than it sounds. I asked myself: "What can I do differently? Do I really want to follow the same path as everyone else?"

I only started to apply myself at the start of high school. I read about some of the top academic achievers (who were in Grade 12/ matric) at the time. People revered them. It was then that I truly realized that achieving a top academic position was something that I wanted to achieve. I needed to work hard. That was non-negotiable.

In Primary school; I never performed as well as I hoped to, academically. I eventually understood that it was a crucial time for, "ironing out my mistakes," as my Dad would say.

I will never forget the moment when the rankings for our grade were announced for the first term of our first year of high school. The people who usually performed well, in primary school, had their names called out. Suddenly, my name was called out as the second top achiever in the grade. My heart skipped a beat. It was one of my favorite memories from school. Eventually, I did reach the top position. I remained in the top three spots, throughout high school. I craved the feeling of being at the top. This relentless innate drive for success spurred me on to greater heights. Eventually, I was ranked as the third top private school student in my province-KwaZulu Natal. My twin brother was the top student. After many years I have learned to appreciate that this drive for success is not just the result of, "good genes," (which is assumed by many). It is the product of years of endeavor and adapting to any challenge. I feel that anyone can do this with enough trial and error as well as unrelenting determination.

Competition for university acceptance is fierce. Nelson R. Mandela School of medicine, UKZN, is no exception. You have to perform well academically if you want to be a doctor. People won't trust you to save their kidney if they don't trust you with basic arithmetic. During our first year, we learned that all medical professionals should obtain a high level of competency in 6 important areas: Patient care; medical knowledge; professionalism; systems-based practice; practice-based learning; interpersonal and communication skills (that's a mouthful). In this book; I recall important experiences that shaped me as a medical student and developed my appreciation for the beauty of our work. I also hope to elucidate the world of medicine for others-to leave a breadcrumb trail for those who wish to explore our noble profession.

INTERPERSONAL AND COMMUNICATION SKILLS

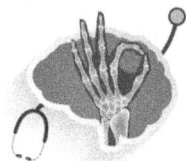

"The art of medicine consists in amusing the patient while nature cures the disease."

— *VOLTAIRE*

ATTITUDE

I f you think you know everything, med school will hit you like a sledgehammer. Here are some basic survival tips. Having the right attitude and mindset is at the core of any successful academic pursuit. Once you display the personality, tact, and work ethic of a top student; motivation and tangible results will likely follow. Many of my friends who wish to study medicine and others who just want to learn more about my line of work have asked me to give them advice. Here are some of the important things that I learned, during my scholastic career, so far. I learned many of these lessons through trial and error, blood, sweat, tears (and other body fluids) and from other people such as my dad, teachers, lecturers, doctors, colleagues, as well as successful medical student vloggers and bloggers from abroad. I owe much to them.

Lawrence Dyche from the Albert Einstein College of Medicine referred to interpersonal skills as, "an essential partner of verbal communication." Core humanistic attitudes (curiosity, caring, and respect) as well as linguistic fluency are important for anybody who wants to study and practice medicine. These core attitudes are developed during our medical training, for us to learn effective interpersonal and communication skills, which help us build better relationships. Your friends and family are going to become even more important when you don a lab coat for the first time.

LONG-TERM THINKING AND OPTIMISM

You've got to think big and you've got to think ahead in this profession. Let's use an example: Studying is a long and tedious task for many. What if it doesn't have to be that way? Pause for 30 seconds. Think to yourself: "Yes, if I study for this test early, I will improve my chances of doing well in the test; which will make me feel so much better later." That mindset spared me a lot of tears. Procrastination may be one of your greatest foes, during high school and medical school. Thinking ahead will help you overcome it. Keeping a thorough record of all your assignments, tests, and projects e.g., through a diary or weekly planner is a good starting point. I use notetaking apps on my phone to quickly jot down things that I need to do for the day. I also do this to record any new words that I learn, which has culminated in a robust lexicon of many of my go-to phrases and words for writing and speaking. Thanks to this method, I now know the meaning of the word: "lexicon…" I have to admit, it's a nice-sounding word.

Staying optimistic in medical school is not always easy (especially if you get a low mark for a test). You will have your good days and your days that could have been better. It took me a long time to get over that feeling of post-test ennui. One of my most important lessons from high school was to GET OVER IT. Medical school will be an even more humbling experience. Every failure is an opportunity for success. One thing that consistently motivated me to study was the thrill of learning something interesting, new, and unusual about medicine. Before I started learning pathology (what can go wrong in a body), I had no idea that some people could be born with a heart outside their body. That's mind-blowing! I think that this curiosity should be cultivated before getting into medical school. It is so much easier to study and understand your textbooks when you are motivated by passion.

Of course, you probably won't be interested in everything that you study. Some of my friends avoided our biochemistry lectures like the plague. I believe that we must strive to find something interesting about every topic that we learn. After all, some people are willing to devote their entire lives to some things that you may think are boring. It can be frustrating to be stuck in a subject that you don't like (let alone an entire university course). The feeling hurts. It feels like you keep reaching dead ends. Dwelling on the issue doesn't help. I realized that it is fine to feel angry or sad, for a short while, if you do not achieve what you work for. But it is important to get over it and move onto the next goal. Channel your frustration into aiming for a better outcome next time or take the time to look at it from a different angle. If you stay positive (and you feel you have worked hard enough to deserve that feeling of optimism); half the battle will be won.

CURIOSITY AND ENJOYMENT

You have to love what you do if you want to survive in our line of work. After our first year at university, our class shrunk to nearly half its size. Can you see yourself working 36 hour shifts and liking it? My brother and I watched countless Simpsons episodes during our teens. Even now we can remember witty lines of dialogue from almost any episode. It's easier to recall one of Homer's hilarious speeches than a paragraph in any dusty old textbook. If you enjoy your studies, you will most likely excel at them and stick through with them until the end. Use incentives to boost your enthusiasm for a subject. My thought process is something like this: "If I ace this test; I will feel great when I see my results. My dad will be proud of me and I will learn something that could somehow be useful to me in my life." Any subject can teach you something useful if you are curious and you enjoy what you learn. I think that this is an essential prerequisite to developing curiosity about patients and their conditions. Patients have a sixth sense that can tell them if you are really interested in what they have to say.

CARING, RESPECT, AND RELATIONSHIPS

It's never a good idea to brave any degree alone…at least that's what my friends tell me. We all have challenging days. We've endured long work hours, broken hearts, tough exams and so much more. In all those instances, I found comfort knowing that there was always someone there to support me. I confide in my brother, my dad, or my aunt whenever I need advice. In the medical profession; it is not uncommon to face multiple stressors daily (long work hours, burnout, emotional and social setbacks…the list goes on). Everyone has different approaches to managing their hidden battles. Mine is talking to the people who are closest to me and writing about my thoughts.

Let me tell you about the Gentlemen's Gazette (formerly known as the Bullet Club). That's the name of a, "student mafia" group that my friends and I started on campus. It started off as a joke (we wanted to emulate the Godfather's sense of style). The joke was that most of us were too friendly to think of killing anyone in cold blood or leave a horse's head on someone's bed. Unexpectedly, the bonds of brotherhood between us grew. Throughout medical school, we convened, on weekends, or during the holidays, to have fun, discuss medical school life, our hobbies, romantic pursuits, braais, food reviews and other lighthearted topics. We often traveled together. Our adventures led us to the Drakensberg, Cape Town, and Qwantani Resort in the Free State…where we were attacked by an ostrich, during a very eventful breakfast. It was a huge bird. We tried to throw fruit at it to chase it away (mostly bananas). Luckily, we survived to tell the hilarious tale. Our many misadventures together strengthened our friendship.

It is comforting to know that other people, in your professional environment, experience similar challenges and successes. Empathy-understanding the feelings of your colleagues and patients-is a product of a caring attitude. In my experience, I have found that the more caring doctors are generally more successful than the less caring ones. You're going to meet nice doctors and mean doctors. Get used to it. Ziegelstein wrote about the importance of social engagement in terms of promoting well-being and avoiding burnout, in medical students and residents. Opportunities to meet students from other disciplines were limited for us. This was largely because of differences in scheduled vacation times, between students from different campuses. The campuses were also really far apart. This also made it a bit harder to meet girls from other campuses…

Despite this, I made great efforts to talk to as many people as I could from both my medical school and other universities (social media deserves much credit for this). Medical students are (stereotypically) not always the most sociable people. Nevertheless, we are expected to work together as part of a united health system. Never underestimate the value of networking and making new friends. My brother and I love throwing big parties. You might be surprised by medical students' tolerance for alcohol. Two heads are better than one. A student in your class could become the minister of health. Why not get to know your colleagues better? Even greeting your colleagues every day goes a long way to establishing a positive rapport with them. It really helps if the nurses like you. They might even change their minds about calling you back in the early hours of the morning to do extra ward work.

The friendships that you form in medical school can have a significant effect on your social and mental wellbeing. During our first year, a sort of social Pangaea happened. Small cliques started to form. We had an interesting mix of students from all over South Africa and Lesotho. At least 6 different languages were spoken in our class. Many people formed small groups because of social preference as well as language and cultural differences amongst students. In our fourth year, we were divided into even smaller groups, when we were assigned to different hospitals. That meant that we had to see the same 15 people in the hospital almost every day from 4th to 6th year. Be on good terms with your colleagues. It makes your life easier, especially if you need them to help you draw blood.

I have made it a personal objective to maintain my friendships and continue to expand my network of interesting contacts. You never know when one of your colleagues could help you learn something amazing and vice versa. This of course extends to your superiors as well. Getting to know my lecturers better, by taking the time to chat with them in the hallways helped me learn about the genetics labs on our campus, which kickstarted my interest in genetics and the basic sciences.

Learn from the strengths of your friends. One of your colleagues might develop skills that might make him/her an amazing cardiologist. Another might become an amazing psychologist. Someone else might be great at computers. The more diverse the skillset in your group, the higher the likelihood that you could create something novel. One of the guys in our friend group was a food reviewer. Through him, I learnt how to critique food for my travel blog. One of the objectives of our, "student mafia group" was to show other medical students that there are a lot of amazing things that they can still do in their spare time, especially if they work with others.

One line that you may often hear from other medical students is, "I'm sorry I couldn't meet you. I'm just really busy." As someone who schedules time for studying, kung fu, piano practice, writing, research, gym training, relaxation, app development, TV presenting, community service, and downtime; I can assure you that there is always enough time for you to do the things that matter to you. If you plan well enough ahead; I feel that there can always be enough time to socialize with your friends and expand your network. I usually leave my Friday nights free to meet with friends for dinner. Even a 5-minute phone call can be a good way to let your friends know that you care for them. It clears the mind and gives you a chance to laugh and reminisce.

There are two sides to every coin. The conflict between medical students, doctors, and patients is a quotidian challenge. Many doctors and students bring their domestic problems to work. Try to avoid this as much as possible. Everyone faces problems, but venting your anger on patients or colleagues will only burn your bridges. Expect to be berated by consultants and supervising doctors for almost anything. I have learned not to take it personally. Some of them will insult you or attack your self-esteem in front of patients and colleagues. Don't let it get to you. They may have problems in their personal lives. They might just be trying to toughen you up. You will grow thicker skin in the wards. Reflect on their constructive criticism, but shrug off any insults. However, you should take action and report colleagues if you feel abused by them. A useful tip that I learned is to politely greet all the health staff in your ward when you arrive at your ward. Remember to smile as well and try to remember their names. Respect will help you build crucial relationships everywhere, especially in medical school and the hospital wards. You may be surprised by how well you will be received by many of your colleagues. Frequently ask if you can help the interns or the doctors as well. They will remember you, which will mean that you will make new friends. Who knows? They could mark you for your clinical examinations someday. You could also learn some great new skills from people in other fields. We're all part of a multidisciplinary team. A nurse from Mahatma Gandhi hospital taught me more about obstetrics than any doctor. She also taught me an interesting curry recipe.

Forging strong positive relationships with your colleagues can open a lot of doors for you. Many of the older doctors and professors in my university knew my brother, and me because my dad made a good impression, when he was a medical student. Good manners, respect, and attentive listening skills have also helped me a great deal, in the wards. Extending one's hand to fellow doctors for a handshake usually disarms and impresses them. Many studies show that good medical communication and interpersonal skills are beneficial for doctors as well as their patients and colleagues. How you manage your relationships in your personal and professional lives is critical for delivering optimum care. Never forget this.

Medical school is humbling. Most of the students in my year were the top students in their respective schools. The students at the top are not invincible. The best students in your year are just like everyone else. You may ask: "How do they do it? Surely, they study every hour of the day? Do they even have a life?" More often than not, they succeed because they have a life. A well-balanced life is important for excelling in university. You don't have to conform and just be a bookworm. Be interesting. Many of my friends who perform well academically attest to this. You will probably meet many students who will vie for coveted academic positions or rankings. Fostering healthy competition between you and your colleagues will improve your academic performance immensely. Help your colleagues, when they are in need. Assist them, when they need your advice. Congratulate them when they do well, honestly. Look them straight in the eye. Swallow your pride. Give him/her a firm handshake and say, "Well done." Do not relent, even when you perform better than them. Keep finding smarter ways to study and practice your art and keep encouraging your colleagues to improve. It helps everyone.

Of course, it is incredibly helpful to make friends outside of medicine as well. I owe much to my friends, both locally and abroad, who taught me so many incredible lessons that have shaped me into the person I am today. By meeting people from all walks of life, my views of the world have been broadened. Thanks to them, I have explored different fields that have helped not just my medical career, but many other aspects of my life. By making friends in the TV and film industry, I improved my public speaking skills and started TV presenting work, which also helped my clinical oral presentation skills. I have always felt that entertainment is one of the best ways to educate people. My entry into the entertainment industry began fortuitously after I created a series of online comedy skits to educate my friends and family about the COVID-19 pandemic, which started during my 5th year of medical school. (In case you haven't noticed, I love humor). A local TV show hired me to interview different people such as victims of violent crimes, prostitution, and gender-based violence (which deepened my understanding of social determinants of health in my community). By making friends in app development and software engineering, I designed an app as well, improved my coding skills for my genetics research, and started a small business.

Branch out and meet people from all walks of life. I came across a beggar outside a McDonald's with a few of my classmates, after a late night of partying. The delirious man claimed that he "knew everything." Somehow, he knew the admission criteria for Harvard university medical school, which he shouted at us from outside the restaurant. None of us saw that coming.

Making friends through my travels has shown me how different people approach health in different parts of the world. By forming new connections in different ways, the chances of creating something novel become greater and you have more fun and create amazing memories.

3

BALANCE

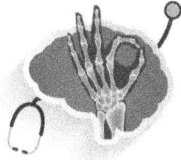

> *"Your hand opens and closes, opens and closes. If it were always a fist or always stretched open, you would be paralyzed. Your deepest presence is in every small contracting and expanding, the two as beautifully balanced and coordinated as birds' wings."*

> *— JALALUDDIN RUMI, THE ESSENTIAL RUMI*

Let me give you some context about life in medical school. I will also share some tips that will help you survive in this melting pot. A universally accepted stereotype in high school is that the top students are isolated bookworms with little else to offer, except an astounding ability to recall facts from textbooks and apply them in a test situation. This couldn't be further from the truth. Throughout my travels, I have had chance encounters with several young and successful intellects. One of them is the world's youngest actuary (who inspired me to start writing this book many years ago), The majority of them have a common trait: Versatility. Why put all your eggs in one basket?

I was privileged to have a caring dad, who encouraged me to try new things. Every Saturday morning, during our primary school years, my brother and I tried some new activity with him. Diving, golf, tennis…you name it. Despite the protests of our exhausted 10-year-old selves we tagged along, half-conscious. At the time, I didn't realize how important it was to start broadening my skill set at a young age.

Many people have the preconceived notion that medical school leaves little time for anything besides rigorous studying. Developing new skills, that are unrelated to medicine, reminded me that there are other ways to invest time and effort to become a better scholar and human being. It is helpful to think: "What do I want to achieve at the end of medical school?" Sure, you may graduate…but so will hundreds of other people. Attaining a degree, for many, is the product of years of toil and learning. This is an incredible accolade. But what will set you apart? The psychologist, Robert Ornstein, proposed the theory that our perception of the speed of time is greatly affected by the amount of information (especially new information) that is available to the mind for absorption and processing. If you have more interesting experiences, time seems to pass more slowly, which will help you remember your student years better. Developing new skills in your spare time is one of the best ways to do this. Do not fret. You might scoff at this seemingly obvious tip. You might wonder, "how will I ever have time for anything else when I already have enough coursework?" Trust me. I felt the same way for many years. Whenever I feel this way; I remember a basic physics principle that I learnt in high school: "The coefficient of static friction is always greater than the coefficient of kinetic friction on any given surface." I think this principle applies to learning any new skill. You always need more energy to get something started. It gets easier from there.

There are some amazing people who studied with me. One girl became a successful Youtuber. A few others started their small businesses, by selling medical equipment. They hustled and reaped the rewards. It is very easy to become institutionalized. If your life only revolves around studying or work; you might find yourself sucked into a repetitive orbit. When you eventually finish high school or your university degree; ask yourself:" What did I achieve during those years?" Try it out on somebody you know. I woke up, one morning and pondered over it.

6 years of your life is precious time. Make the most of it.

My twin brother and I started playing the piano in grade 1. Even now, I make time to play the piano every day and learn a new piece. We tried competitive swimming; golf, tennis, and table tennis. Eventually, we also started kung fu training. Studying medicine seems like a full-time commitment. On some days, we started at 8:00am and ended at 10:00pm, during hospital intakes. Trust me. You get used to it. I discovered that it is exceptionally important to remember that people will make time for things that matter to them. After a 4-hour ward round in a hospital, I too, long for the sweet embrace of my bed. Thoughts of postponing any one of my extracurricular activities do cross my mind. We're human. There are days when we just want to relax. I realized that all those extra skills complemented my studies greatly. You can learn something from any skill that you hone. For example, I developed a much greater appreciation for the action of different muscle groups after learning different stances from my kung fu training and by practicing my golf swing. The exercise and extra time to clear my head helped my studies a lot as well. Diversifying your skillset is incredibly useful and can be help you in unexpected ways. Learning Spanish helped me answer a tough question on an exam once, because I recognized the Latin root of the word.

It's impossible to work 24/7. Taking a break every Friday afternoon and evening, to go out for a movie or to meet friends; or to play video games, helps me calm down at the end of a tough week. I love taking strolls along the beach. I have realized that there is a critical difference between resting and doing nothing. If you're going to relax-do it with intention and without guilt. That's a common feeling that many of my colleagues complained about. If you schedule your time well enough, then you will also be able to find enough time to study and relax well. There should be no reason for an excuse. This is easier said than done of course and there were times when my schedule did not always work out as planned. Enjoy your downtime and study extra to balance it out. If you can't accommodate changes in your schedule immediately, then reschedule them. Make time for yourself and the people you care about and the things that you enjoy doing. My dad always told me: "Work hard and party hard." If you do either one half-heartedly, there is a good chance that you will feel unsatisfied by both. Some medics can party really hard...

My typical daily high school schedule was something like this: 1. 6:30 am (wake up; shower; brush my teeth; change into my school uniform and eat breakfast (oats with some fruit). 2. 8:00 am-2:30 pm (school classes) 3. 3:00 pm-4:00 pm (lunch and an afternoon nap) 4. 4:30 pm-7:00 pm (extra tuition classes, tennis, table tennis or golf) 5. 7:30 pm-12:30 am (homework, revision, studying and dinner). It was like clockwork. I am sure that there are many students whose schedules are even busier than mine. Many students who I have met make excuses like." I don't have enough time" or," I feel so tired." I felt the same way at one point. I no longer make those excuses. Exercise helped. Starting an exercise routine was extremely challenging during the first 2-3 months. It got much easier over time. Exercise is also very important for your mental health. You need to take care of yourself. Sitting at a desk all day won't cut it.

I maintained this schedule throughout my medical school years as well. I needed to make a few changes, however, when we started 4th year (our first year in the school of clinical medicine).

It helps to maintain a consistent schedule. There will be days when you might feel really tired and just don't want to work. There will also be unpredictable changes in your schedule. That's okay. Adapt. I still fit in at least one hour of training at the gym, Kung-fu practice, or piano practice into each day. It keeps me sane...and I am a healthier person because of it.

When people ask me:" Do you even have a life outside medical school?" I now say: "Of course. How can you not?."

At the end of medical school, most people will graduate with their degree. This in itself is an incredible achievement. But what if you can go beyond that? Everybody else in your class will most likely achieve the same as well. I reiterate this point. What will set you apart? There is no one-size-fits-all answer to this question. From, my experience, we all must find interests that inspire and motivate us. By developing new skills, interests, and hobbies, my medical career improved and became much more wholesome and enjoyable. I am a strong advocate for the idea that broadening our interests broadens our vocational horizons.

By seeking balance in our lives (physically, emotionally, socially and spiritually) we become healthier people. It's even part of the World Health Organization definition of health for goodness sake! If we are healthier people we can help others become healthier too.

4

THE PRECLINICAL YEARS

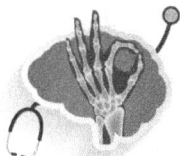

"The important thing is that you've got a strong foundation before you start to try to save the world or help other people."

— *RICHARD BRANSON*

A h! The preclinical years. We all have to start somewhere. These are fun years. There is a good chance that you will have a lot of free time. Use it wisely. I reflect on some of the most salient experiences from my preclinical years of medical school. I believe that these experiences are critical for becoming a compassionate and competent doctor. Michael S. Kavic lists and explains 6 core competencies that all physicians should master: 1. Interpersonal and Communication Skills-skills that allow for effective information exchange and collaboration with patients, their families, and other health care professionals; 2. Application of medical knowledge about established and constantly changing biomedical, clinical, epidemiological, and social-behavioral sciences, to patient care; 3. Patient care-Compassion when treating patients; 4. Practice-based learning and improvement-Investigating and evaluating how one cares for patients, how one uses scientific evidence, and how one improves patient care. 5. Professionalism-commitment to carrying out professional responsibilities, adhering to ethical principles, and being sensitive to a diverse patient population. 6. Systems-based practice-understanding that you are part of a bigger picture, in a health system. That's a lot of things to work on over 6 hears. I feel that I developed the last 3 competencies the most during my clinical years (years 4-6).

Learning medical knowledge, starts mainly in the preclinical years (years 1-3 in South Africa) and is developed through clinical experience during the clinical years. But remember to have fun during these years! I recall some good times laughing with friends at our small cafeteria on campus or playing table tennis with my colleagues. Whenever the table tennis board collapsed, we bolstered it with boxes of condoms...which were abundant because of the many HIV awareness campaigns that took place on campus.

When my colleagues and I first started medical school, we couldn't have looked wetter behind the ears. We no longer needed to wear school uniforms, so many of us chose to wear the most comfortable clothes we had-jeans, T-shirts, sweatpants. I think back on those days fondly. It was a liberating time for us. We were the new kids on the block, in a new and exciting environment. It was a dream come true. Merely being accepted into Nelson R. Mandela School of medicine, one of the most exclusive medical schools in South Africa, was a reason to celebrate.

The first year was a steep learning curve. We needed to take care of a lot of boring admin work like registration and organizing payment of our tuition fees. In addition to that, we had to find out where each department was. Our student executive committee organized a scavenger hunt to help us navigate our way through the labyrinth of hallways on campus. Even today, I still get lost on campus. Every day, I find new rooms. There was even a rumor that there was a dark secret room on "floor zero" beneath our dissecting hall. Some of my friends told me that it was filled with buckets of blood. It could have just been paint...maybe. I joked that if anyone could reason their way through the complicated university registration website and the campus hallways, they were automatically smart enough to qualify for graduation from our medical school.

Our syllabus for the first 3 years was divided into 2 main subjects. One subject was basic foundational sciences (which included topics that formed the basis of our understanding of medicine, such as physics, chemistry, anatomy, physiology, biochemistry, clinical methods, and pharmacology, to name a few). The second main subject was Becoming a Professional (which covered topics such as medical ethics, professionalism in healthcare, and public health). We affectionately referred to these subjects as BFS and BAP respectively. Every year, we also needed to complete community service projects. The 2 main community service projects that we were required to complete by the end of our third year of medical school were called The Making a Difference Project and the Selectives Project.

Most of our material was taught in the form of didactic lectures and tutorials in a large lecture venue (L7). It feels exciting at first, to be seated in a large, tiered room, with so many top students and to be lectured by local legends in the fields of science and medicine. Despite that, I am sure that all of us fell asleep in at least one lecture. I remember how nervous I felt whenever I was asked to answer questions in front of the entire class. Everyone turned their heads to look at whoever dared to raise his/her hand. It didn't take us long to realize that this fear was unreasonable. We were there to learn and make mistakes, regardless of what other people thought about us. Now my brother and I aren't afraid to ask questions at any time. We learned that it is better to ask a question than to remain silent and not know the answer. I don't know how many times I've answered questions incorrectly in front of my class.

We started to realize that the days were passing much faster than they did in high school. We were no longer writing tests every week and we hardly did any assignments. We wrote our tests approximately every 6 weeks. If we performed well for the tests, we were exempted from writing exams. That was one clear incentive for working hard. There was this newfound freedom that we were all relishing. There was no-one to watch over us and berate us for not doing homework or not submitting an assignment. It was all up to us. This is a double-edged sword. Those who relied too strongly on teachers and tutors for motivation were taught a harsh lesson. Medical school demanded that we work responsibly and show initiative to learn our course material.

Lectures usually started at 8:00 am and ended around 2:00-4:00 pm (when many of us were half asleep). Many of the lecturers just read-off the lecture slides, which meant that most students chose to optimize their learning time by picking and choosing which lectures to attend. My brother and I still chose to attend as many lectures as possible. At least we could learn the lecture beforehand and ask questions. My advice for students is to attend the lectures that you feel will give you the best output for your time invested. If a lecturer takes 2 hours to teach something that you could learn well in half the time, then just learn it yourself.

Our dissecting hall (DH) sessions and clinical methods training were scheduled during early morning and early afternoon hours. Our first dissecting hall visit was unforgettable. Many of us were filled with a sense of excitement…and hesitation. For many of us, Grey's Anatomy and CSI were our only references for cutting dead bodies. I had never seen a corpse before visiting

DH. The same could be said for many of my other colleagues…
hence our hesitation.

The first thing that hit us as we stepped into DH was the
overwhelming odor of formalin-a chemical that helps preserve
cadavers. It lingers in the air and you smell of it for the rest of
the day. We all gagged simultaneously. Eventually, it turned into
a mildly pungent smell as we became desensitized to it.

Rows of bodies were covered in fabric and lined up on metal
tables. They were illuminated by bright overhead lights. We
were divided into groups of 5 and bodies were assigned to us.
My hand trembled as I uncovered our cadaver for the first time.
It was the body of an elderly white male. His eyes stared back at
me listlessly-locked in an eternal gaze. His most striking feature
was his papery skin. He closely resembled a mummy. My entire
group was silent.

I looked closely at his deep black pupils and wondered what
things he had seen during his long life. I lowered my head as a
sign of respect for this unknown man who donated his body to
science. Throughout our first 2 years of medical school, my
group became closely acquainted with him. We cut open his
body and held his heart, his lungs, and his abdominal organs. It
felt surreal. We held parts of him that he had never seen, even
though he relied on them daily, for survival. It felt like finding
out a secret about a person, even before they knew about it,
themselves. Those dissecting hall sessions greatly deepened my
respect for the human body. It is a work of infinite beauty and
genius. The fact that all the organ systems work harmoniously to
help us live is a phenomenon of infinite complexity. Everything
seems to be so perfectly positioned in the body. Even walking, a
seemingly simple act that many of us take for granted requires
complex co-ordination between many muscles and nerves
working in concert with each other. Understandably, learning all
the nerves, muscles, measurements and anatomical structures in

our anatomy atlases was going to take a long time. Distinguishing one nerve from another was, notoriously, one of our most challenging tasks in DH (they all look like spaghetti). Anatomy became even more relevant, in my clinical years, when I was required to examine patients and remember the locations of different organs that were affected by different pathologies. We studied specimens of every organ system in the DH: brains, lungs, hearts, stomachs, pancreases, uteruses, penises, you name it. There were even small organs and embryos floating in small tubes all around the DH.

Our anatomy tutors supervised us. We made the necessary cuts, as recommended in the book: Grant's dissector. I have to say, I felt really powerful holding a scalpel for the first time. It's an energizing feeling that makes you think: "Wow, I'm doing something that a surgeon would do." I was also surprised by how heavy a cadaver can be. Turning the body over to make incisions on the back, could only be done with the coordinated effort of our entire group of 5.

When we completed our final anatomy exam, we were overcome with relief. Long hours in a room filled with formalin and cadavers tend to make one hungry and exhausted-especially the afternoon sessions. We left the DH for the last time, a bit unceremoniously. But I couldn't help but bow my head once more as a sign of respect to the body of the elderly man on the metal table who taught me so much, without ever saying a word.

During our clinical skills sessions, we learned many of the procedural and examination skills that we would need for our clinical years. We were divided into small groups and assigned to different clinical skills tutors in our skills lab, which was a fairly large room filled with different clinical skills training equipment (like CPR dummies and defibrillators). We were first taught to take histories from patients (which is arguably our most important clinical skill). Many skilled doctors attest that most of the information required to make a clinical diagnosis can be elicited from history alone. This meant that we needed to ask patients important, and often personal questions about their health (which includes questions about their symptoms, background history, and social history). Our clinical skills teacher was fond of reminding us that doctors need to be good actors. For the first 2 years of medical school, we practiced among our colleagues. Eventually, we learned to take much more specific and nuanced histories that are more relevant to patients with specific medical conditions, such as sexual histories. Asking complete strangers personal questions demands that we overcome shyness and personal prejudices. Yes, you will have to ask questions about people's sex lives.

The head of our clinical skills department was the mother of one of my friends from high school. Thanks to her protocols for examining patients, she helped many students improve their confidence in their clinical skills. She created step-by-step recommendations for examining patients' different body systems, like the cardiovascular examination or the respiratory examination. We needed to know a logical sequence for touching and assessing different parts of the body. We also needed to perform some really sensitive exams. In my 4th year, I was asked to perform a prostate exam on a man in his 60s. It was an interesting learning experience…that was probably more uncomfortable for the patient. Our trauma lecturers like to remind us that we must be comfortable with, "sticking fingers in every orifice." Many of us needed time to grasp the concept of using protocols and algorithms for approaching clinical thinking and clinical examinations. It makes sense. After observing many skilled physicians in different hospitals, I have come to realize that reaching a diagnosis rarely involves a sudden flash of intuitive lightning. More often than not it is a process that requires a flow of thought-gradually accumulating evidence from history and examination findings until a most likely diagnosis is considered. Our clinical skills lecturers often likened doctors to detectives because of this. Welcome to the club, Sherlock.

It was fascinating to see how certain students excelled at one examination technique over the other. Some were better at hearing heart sounds. Others were better at feeling for and describing masses in the abdomen. This is another example of the immense diversity of medicine and the people who work in the field. I have often said to my friends that there is a medical discipline for everyone. If you like photography, you might like ophthalmology or radiology. If you like video games and fine motor skills, surgery might be right up your alley. If strength training and sports appeal to you, sports medicine or orthopedics may be the job for you. The options are vast, which is another reason why I love medicine.

Of course, mastering these clinical skills is a different story entirely. It requires lifelong commitment. Initially, listening to heart sounds was challenging for me. It was hard to time the "lub-dub" sound which is caused by the opening and closure of different heart valves. Eventually, in my 4th year, our class received a lecture from a leading cardiology professor from one of our quaternary/research hospitals (Inkosi Albert Luthuli Hospital). Then, everything made sense to me, but only after much trial and error. Making the correct diagnosis feels like an adrenaline rush.

Many people tell new medical students that the first 2 years of medical school are easy and relaxed because much of our time is spent learning basic concepts that are similar to what we learned in high school. For many students, this may be true. For others, it may be more challenging. That is another important lesson that I learned from medical school: I learnt to take the advice of more senior students with a pinch of salt. Everybody responds to different subjects in medicine differently. We have our strengths and weaknesses and so do others. One should not start any new subject in medicine with a bias, created by anyone else who already did the subject. My approach was to do my best and keep improving. I needed to forge my own path. You will forge a different path entirely.

In my 2nd and 3rd year, we started learning basic pathology and systems specific subjects such as the respiratory system, the cardiovascular system, the gastrointestinal system, the central nervous system, endocrinology...and many other words ending with" ology." Basically, we needed to learn what can go wrong in the human body...which is a lot.

For me, this was my first taste of what medical school coursework was really about. We were given reams of pages of notes and expected to learn them in a short time. We were expected to know all the diseases that can commonly affect almost every organ system. It took me a while to realize the importance of thinking long-term when studying those subjects. It is easy to become overwhelmed by the sheer volume of course material. You could probably bench press some of the heavier textbooks. Even in the clinical years, doctors still ask us to recall information from our preclinical years, which is fair game. They are called basic foundational sciences for a reason. They form the foundation of our medical school knowledge. The foundation must be strong before one can build upon it. Yes, we must aim to perform well for one's tests and exams, but we should ask ourselves the question: "How will we use new information? And where does this new information fit in the bigger scheme of things?" When I realized the relevance of what we were learning, everything made much more sense and I was more invested in learning about it. I recall one instance, during my 3rd year when I was paging through a neuroanatomy textbook in our university library- a cool and dusty place where my dad studied many years before me. I made sure that I took the time to learn the different nerve pathways, which are long and can get complicated. For my final 4th-year internal medicine exam, I was required to assess a patient with a stroke-a case that requires a thorough understanding of basic neuroanatomy. You never know when you will need your knowledge of the basic sciences to answer clinical questions... therefore you must know it well. Constant spaced repetition and active recall of information yield better results than cramming. My Kung Fu instructor once told me that a master is just someone who knows the basics extremely well. I agree with him. Everything else in medicine stems from the basics. Even in our 5th and 6th-year exams, many of our examiners tested our knowledge of basic sciences. Never underestimate the importance of working hard during the preclinical years. Improving my understanding of the basic sciences is something that I intend to continue doing, for the rest of my life. Even the greatest diagnosticians can reason everything down to the basics.

This knowledge carries us into the clinical years-an entirely different experience that tests not just our knowledge and clinical skills, but every part of our being. It was during those years, when I truly felt that I started to develop the final 3 competencies that every medical student should master, before they graduate, according to Michael S. Kavic.

In my experience, these last 3 competencies: professionalism, patient care, practice-based learning, and systems-based care, like all the other competencies, are inextricable-you can't just become good at one, without becoming good at all the others.

One experiences a myriad of emotions during the different undergraduate clinical rotations-joy, heartbreak, anger towards a harsh consultant...the list goes on. These rotations, which can last anywhere from 6 weeks to 12 weeks, change you as a person. Thousands of hours are spent at the bedside and in the operating theatre. Blood will be drawn. Tutorials will be attended. Friendships will be forged in the wards-those democracies of appearance. You will see patient gowns, devastated and relieved complexions, tubes and IV lines. In this crucible, where life is renewed and taken away; we witness some of life's most beautiful and crushing moments. These places are autoclaves for the soul, where pressure, high patient caseloads, and low resources purify us-they force us to abandon or challenge our vices, to help others. These experiences are life-changing and profound. In my anecdotes, I try to capture this profoundness...the clinical years is where the real adventure begins.

5

PEDIATRICS

A new milestone

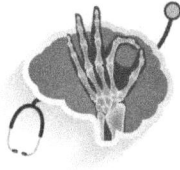

"In Greek, our word for play is paidia and the word for education is paideia, and it is very natural and right that these words should be entangled at the root, together with our word for children, paides, which gave you your words pedagogy and pediatrician."

— *REBECCA GOLDSTEIN*

Pediatrics was my first rotation in the school of clinical medicine. It felt like an appropriate block with which to start my clinical career. Pediatrics is a branch of medicine that deals with children and their diseases. Children are curious and constantly learning...but they are vulnerable as well, much like we were, as new members of the healthcare team. We had some clinical exposure during our 3rd year (known as the clinical methods block) which involved us visiting hospitals once every week, to practice our basic history taking and examination skills on actual patients. It was a big step-up from practicing with our fellow students or on CPR dummies (which look very creepy). Just as children learn new important milestones for the rest of their lives, so too did we have to learn critical new clinical skills which are important for the rest of our medical careers. It was a steep learning curve. We were expected to know all our basic examinations for pediatrics (namely the chest, abdomen, neurological and general exams). The general exam (which involves quickly looking at a patient and recording their vital signs) helps us quickly assess the patient's general wellbeing. We were also required to learn new clinical assessment tools that are specific to the discipline of pediatrics (like growth measurements and children's developmental milestones). Our consultants expected us to do this within a very narrow time frame (5 weeks), much to their frustration and ours.

We were examined during our 6th week of the block. In addition to that, we needed to write 2 patient reports and study all our lecture notes. No pressure. It wasn't long before we realized that this would become the norm during our clinical years. It was a far cry from our preclinical years when we were required to just write multiple-choice exams or spotter exams (which is an assessment that requires us to identify anatomical structures on human cadavers/specimens in the DH). I recall something that my dad told me that he learned in medical school. Any medical student who tells you that they only started studying/working for an exam the night before actually writing it…is probably lying. Hard work is a given in medical school. That concept was beaten into us by the consulting doctors who expected us to know everything about pediatrics within 6 weeks. Throughout my years of medical school, I have learned that doctors come in all flavors. The spectrum of their teaching styles is broad. Some focus more on inflating their ego and reinforcing the hierarchy in the hospital. Others teach with care, compassion, and love for their students. We all preferred the latter. But an important lesson was that we needed to roll with the punches and not take any of their aggressive remarks to heart. We needed to achieve the results that we desired. As long as the doctors helped us learn what we needed to know, many of us didn't mind their rants. We wanted to examine patients so well that the doctors couldn't grill us.

Childhood is fraught with challenges and dangers. Many of them help us grow into stronger people and adapt to change. Pediatrics is no different.

We attended lectures on Mondays. The rest of the week was spent in hospital wards. The image of rows of rusty patient beds and the green linoleum hospital floors was burned into our minds. Our entire class was divided into smaller groups, which were allocated to different disciplines and hospitals. I was sent to Addington Hospital-along Durban's beautiful North beach.

Durban, my home city, is famous for its beaches (some have dubbed it the Miami of South Africa). The water is warm all year and the city boasts an impressive beach promenade, The Golden Mile, that extends from the Moses Mabhida Stadium (where several soccer world cup matches took place in 2010) all the way to our bustling harbor. I woke up on the morning of my first hospital day in mid-January-one of the hottest times of the year. I was raring to go.

Finding the hospital required me to navigate the hot and congested streets that snake alongside Durban's North beachfront, which is lined with luxury hotels. There is so much energy there. Cyclists, joggers, pedestrians, frenetic street-performers, colorful rickshaw drivers, street hawkers, and pigeons mingle freely. Some of the medical students soak in this vibrant atmosphere, during break times. I enjoyed eating my lunch on the dunes or visiting the beachside restaurants whenever I had a few minutes to spare before our clinical tutorials. You could get amazing burgers and milkshakes there. The hospital commutes and those blissful moments on the beach reminded me how much I love my city.

My phone alarm usually pulled me back to reality, whenever it was time to examine patients or attend a clinical teaching session, which involved us presenting our patient reports to senior doctors. Addington hospital is a huge building that was meant to be the largest hotel in Durban many years ago. Decades of exposure to the sea breeze and infrequent maintenance have led to a slow decline in the building's facilities and equipment (the elevators are often out of order). The hospital may have seen better days, but it continues to serve a large portion of our city's patients and it has been going strong for many years. On some days I jogged up the 12 flights of stairs, to get to the pediatric wards. The burst of energy helped prepare me for my day. I befriended one of the interns who told me about a secret elevator, that was used mostly by the cleaning staff. At least that was another option. Sometimes, it shuddered to a halt, when I was in it. It makes the heart skip a beat.

Most of our time was spent in the pediatric wards examining children or in the clinics, where we took growth measurements and helped with minor procedures. The wards were colorful and decorated with stickers of Disney characters. Many of the children and their families were foreigners from neighboring countries and other parts of Africa. I managed to impress one of my consultants during a ward round by explaining why newborns don't tend to be affected by sickle cell anemia (which is a disease that causes the red blood cells to become sickle-shaped, instead of the normal biconcave disk shape). It is a fairly common condition among patients from certain African countries-where having the disease can protect people against getting malaria, to some degree. I even met a patient from Western Africa with the condition. He is the first 7-year-old I've met who knows the word: "hydroxyurea" (one of the drugs used to help manage the condition). I gave him a high-five because I was so impressed.

To be honest, I don't think that adults give children enough credit. I love talking to children as well as adults. Children generally want to find out things and they aren't afraid to ask for help. That makes them fun to talk to because many of them are genuinely interested when I try to teach them things. Whenever my aunts asked me to watch over their babies, I used to cradle them in my arms and start talking about deep philosophical concepts (even if they were too young to talk or understand what I was saying). They usually stared blankly at me. It was funny and it made my aunts laugh most of the time.

I owe a lot to my dad for satisfying my thirst for knowledge as a child. I remember that he owned a set of medical journals, which he usually left open on his desk. Even though I didn't understand most of the contents of the journals at the time, I wanted to feel important and learned like the people who wrote the journals. I paged through them when I was in primary school. That is probably the earliest memory I have of loving medicine and science.

Our emergency medicine teacher is a qualified paramedic. She taught us CPR and resuscitation techniques from our 1st to 5th year of medical school. She became famous at our university for her matter-of-fact no-nonsense style of teaching. If a patient collapsed in front of us, we needed to know what to do. There was no room for error. She had many years of experience resuscitating people. She was fond of telling us that children tend to respond very well to resuscitation efforts. They are strong and resilient. But they are also vulnerable…

During our medical ethics lessons, we were taught how to recognize child abuse and how to respond accordingly. Children are involved in many ethically challenging situations such as: "What to do if a child is a Jehovah's Witness, but he/she needs a blood transfusion?" or, "What do you do if you suspect child abuse as the cause of multiple bone fractures in a child?" Our government sets out guidelines for addressing these scenarios. Every day as students, we are reminded that we will deal with these ethical challenges in practice and we need to know how to react to them if we want to protect vulnerable members of society.

In Durban, there is a stark contrast between the rich and the poor. The city center has seen its fair share of urban decay. I live in a comfortable suburb, where sports cars are commonplace and some families own more than one palatial mansion. All it takes is a 10-minute drive towards the city center (known by the locals as "town") to see numerous beggars or hawkers trying to eke out a living while wearing little more than rags. It is a heart-wrenching sight. Many of the beggars are children. Many of them roam outside Addington hospital. They remind me of how closely social conditions and health are intertwined and why it is so important that we improve our social situation if we want to end the cycle of poverty that keeps children begging on the streets and ending up in our hospitals.

This is the first article that I wrote, during the first clinical rotation of my 4th year of medical school, to capture some of my more memorable moments from the pediatrics block.

THE SURVIVORS OF 13A

The gargantuan edifice of Addington hospital boldly faces Durban's North Beach. The monolithic structure is hard to miss. I spent 6 weeks there. On my first day at the hospital, a security guard at the entrance gave my bag a cursory glance to confirm that I was not carrying any landmines (which were drawn on warning posters, opposite the cafeteria for some reason). Stepping into that hospital feels like a slow rewinding of time. Much of the hospital has seemingly not changed since the 1960s. In the 1940s a 4500-ton merchant ship was wrecked close to North beach. The hospital (which was incomplete at the time) admitted those who survived. During my month of training at Addington, I saw people drowning...figuratively. I met people who clung to their families and loved ones as the tempest of illness and disease tried to dash hope against the rocks of North Beach...in the pediatric wards.

A striking feature about Addington hospital is the proximity of the children's hospital outpatient department (or CHOPD for short) to the mortuary. The starkness of the opposition of what those places represent (the start of life and the end of life) lead me to question how people view illness at both life's inception and conclusion.

Atul Gawande, one of my favorite physician writers, suggests in his novel, "Being Mortal" that the elderly choose to pursue new ambitions, friendships, power, and goals less aggressively than younger people, in favor of appreciating what they already have. Some reach an acceptance of their mortality. Others, along with their family members rage mightily against the dying of the light and opt for treatments (many of which may be useless) to grasp at even a razor-thin chance of survival.

What happens to a child, under the age of 12 years, who is faced with a similar situation? How many of us even ask the children how they feel about their conditions?

After spending a few weeks in ward 13A (the pediatric ward) I learned ways to befriend children. Blowing up a latex glove like a balloon (and drawing a smiley face on it) was a great way to endear myself to the younger kids. Dangling a small plush doll above the babies allowed me a few precious seconds to distract them and sneak in a quick abdominal exam. Some of the children are very eager to be examined and affectionately imitate auscultation techniques when they grasp a stethoscope. It is an adorable sight.

Some studies predict that mortality is only understood by children between the ages of 4-6. How do younger children understand disease? How many doctors avoid explaining the idea of mortality to children, out of fear of scaring both the children and their mothers? One of our 2-year-old patients was isolated, to prevent her from spreading multiple drug-resistant tuberculosis. She cried constantly and begged for anyone to enter the room and play with her, even though, we could not. I could only imagine the emotional pain that she felt, as we observed her, from behind a closed door.

The scene of a mother sitting at the bedside of her ailing child in 13A, for a week or more, on a moth-eaten couch is not an uncommon sight. It is both a heartwarming and heart-wrenching image that strongly reminds me of Sandro Botticelli's: "Madonna of the Book." Except in our scenario, the book is the: "Road to Health Chart" -a book which helps mothers track the growth and health of their babies, along with their vaccinations. The mothers are the paragon of devotion, tenderness, and love for their children. I took a history from a mother, who was seated in the ward for 12 consecutive agonizing days, to tend to her child. Her child was diagnosed with cerebral palsy- a condition marked by impaired muscle coordination (spastic paralysis) and/or other disabilities, typically caused by damage to the brain before or at birth. She risked losing her job by taking so much time off work. But she was willing to risk everything to stay by her child's side.

Several American studies on mothers in pediatric wards suggest that mothers tend to take very proactive approaches to decision-making regarding their children's health (e.g., reading online sources and talking to other mothers whose children have similar conditions). I saw this very often in 13A. They spoke among each other and formed friendships. Talking about problems with others helps. They bonded out of desperation.

Many of my colleagues and I were asked: "Is my child dying?" This is often a very difficult question to answer. Oftentimes, many of us say, that with timely administration of the right treatment, some of the conditions can be cured relatively quickly. But what do you say about a patient with a terminal illness? Despite our great progress in medical science, we still don't know everything. Death can be unpredictable. Even if the truth hurts, we must be honest with our patients.

A mother started crying, while I clerked her child (who had hydrocephalus of unknown etiology). Hydrocephalus is a concerning condition that can result in swelling of the head (like a balloon being slowly filled with water) She insisted that her child's condition could lead to blindness and possibly death, even though the surgeons stated those complications were unlikely. I did not know what to say to her.

Many studies, throughout the world, suggest that a lack of communication is a significant cause for maternal anxiety, when children are admitted to pediatric wards, especially at the beginning of hospital admission. Medical communication is a great passion of mine. In many cases, explaining a child's condition to his/her mother both calmly and frequently is suggested as an effective way to relieve this anxiety. I observed this while clerking a patient with a rare chromosomal disorder: DiGeorge syndrome. The mother was initially hostile and tried to prevent me from examining her child. Everything I did seemed to inconvenience her. I decided to sit next to her and casually chat about how she felt about her circumstances. After a brief conversation with her, I cracked a joke about the inadequate hospital air conditioning. Seriously, many air conditioners don't work in the public hospitals. Some summer afternoons in Durban feel like being in an oven. She warmed up to me and consented to my clinical assessment of her child. David Rieff, the American fiction writer, and policy analyst, once stated that many doctors speak to patients as if they are children, but without the care that a sensible adult takes in choosing what words to use with a child. We need to change this.

During my time in 13A, I realized that children are surprisingly observant. Their minds are exceptionally malleable, almost molten. They change and adapt to new stimuli more fluidly than adults. I examined a small child with tuberculosis (TB). She made a game out of running from one end of the ward to the other. It is very unstimulating for a child to just sit in bed and stare at the same 4 green walls every day. I admire adults who maintain this highly adaptable child-like mindset. They keep the inner child alive.

Many children don't fully understand their illnesses. Nevertheless, we do our best to empathize with the emotions of the children as well as their families and continue to help as best as we can, through diagnostic mastery, improved communication skills…and maybe a few glove balloons. I feel that the smile of a healthy child, who has been guided back to safe shores, from the pathological brink, is a venerable motivation for the practice of pediatrics.

By the time I finished my pediatrics rotation, it dawned upon me that the smaller members of the human race cannot be treated as small adults. They are an entirely different entity with an incredible capacity for healing and recovery that continues to impress me. Even some children who are born with heart problems can be seen playing happily alongside other children without heart defects.

I have always enjoyed taking the time to talk to children. Their views of the world are often fresh and inquisitive. Many of the children were very interested to see how my stethoscope worked. Some of them even want to become doctors themselves someday. I echo my previous sentiments about the importance of curiosity when learning medicine. Maintaining a childlike fondness for learning new things goes a long way in medical school.

Children also tend to ask for help, without hesitation. A little girl from Addington hospital couldn't reach her food in a drawer. She was probably 5 or 6 years old. Her mother left the ward for a short while. The girl was diagnosed with a type of cancer called Burkitt's lymphoma-which can cause part of the lower face to swell to large sizes in some patients, which was the case in the little girl. I was saddened by the sight of her disease, but happy because I could help her in some small way. She couldn't speak English much. It was noted in her file that she was an immigrant from a country in West Africa. She pointed to a bowl of putu (maizemeal porridge) next to her bed and then gestured to her open mouth. This is a staple meal in many parts of Africa. It was an adorable sight. I felt a caring paternal energy well up inside me. It is a feeling that motivates me to care for others, much like how any father would care for his ailing child. That experience was also a reminder of the importance of learning to ask for help. I have noticed that many health care professionals do not ask for help, because of ego-related reasons. We need to realize that combining our skills maximizes our chances of caring better for our patients. The ego is less important.

I made a special note of remembering my colleagues on our first day of medical school. We were brimming with youthful energy. We were ready to charge headfirst into the healthcare profession. For many, 6 years of late-night studying, assignments, exams, ward work, and working with unrelenting consultants can erode this enthusiasm. Maintaining my child-like curiosity in medical school and beyond has required great strength. It is not always easy to be optimistic when driving home at 10:00 pm from prince Mshiyeni Hospital, along the freeway, after 6 hours of working in a busy medical outpatient department. But, ultimately, it is a choice we make for ourselves. If we want to stay enthusiastic, curious, and optimistic, only we can make that choice.

The survivors of ward 13A have a different way of looking at things. Those kids made an ordinary glove balloon seem fun. They turned something mundane, like walking through a ward, into a game. Even my stethoscope seemed more interesting when they played with it. Doctors like to tell us that children are not small adults, but maybe adults should be more like small children in some ways.

6

GYNECOLOGY

A tale of two mothers

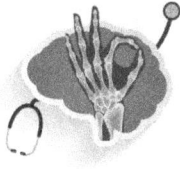

"A male gynecologist is like an auto mechanic who has never owned a car."

— *CARRIE SNOW*

Now let's take things back a bit. Children have to come from somewhere. That brings us to our next discipline of study. At the end of the pediatrics rotation, I wrote a theory exam and completed a clinical examination. My clinical cases included an infant who was born with syphilis (a sexually transmitted infection that was very common even in Victorian times) and an older child with asthma. During the following weekend, we were thrust into our new clinical rotation- gynecology- at Mahatma Gandhi Hospital, in Phoenix-one of the oldest Indian settlements in South Africa. Phoenix is a huge community that conjures up thoughts of hot vibrant Mumbai.

Fortunately, the hospital is very close to where I live, which meant short commutes for my brother and me. The hospital is spread out across a large, dusty, and flat plot of land, dotted with a few saplings. The hospital has seen better days.

Whenever we started a new clinical block, we were required to visit a park home-which is a small building on the hospital property where most of our university administration and orientation takes place. Many park homes were new at the time and contained computer rooms where students could finish their assignments and do research. At least the air conditioners worked there.

For our 6-week rotation, we were instructed to learn our gynecology theory from a South African textbook. Most of our clinical exposure was gained in ward 7A (the gynecology ward), the operating room (where we saw many Caesarean sections), and the labor ward. The hospital was always crowded with patients who carried thick brown files that contained their medical information. There were so many of those files. They filled entire rooms, from floor to ceiling.

There were a few conditions that we were expected to know very well in the wards, such as sexually transmitted infections; HIV/AIDS, miscarriages, and cervical cancer (to name a few). These are bread-and-butter cases that we saw every day in gynecology. We spent most of our time helping with minor procedures like taking blood for lab tests, administering blood transfusions (as many of the women had low blood iron levels), and performing pap smears (which help us determine patients' risks of getting cervical cancer). Taking blood for the first time is not always easy for a student. Sometimes, you can't find the patient's veins at all. You just hope and pray that you succeed on the first attempt. If not, it is wise to ask for a senior doctor to help, instead of jabbing the patient like a frenetic mosquito. It is concerning to think that some at-risk patients, including young women in their 30s, fell through the cracks of our public health system and were not detected during nationwide pap smear campaigns. A pap smear is like a small swab that tells us if a patient is at risk of getting certain types of cervical cancer. Cervical cancer is mainly caused by a virus known as Human Papillomavirus, which can infect the cervix of women. I researched this virus with my research mentor, Dr. Lenine Liebenberg. I then realized how important our research was in understanding the condition and why it tends to cause worse outcomes in some patients with HIV. Translating theoretical knowledge into a clinical setting is an invigorating feeling that reminds me of the importance of supporting ongoing clinical research in our country.

We needed to practice a new style of taking histories from a different kind of patient-adult women. We needed to ask very personal questions-about sexual health, use of contraception, childbirth, and reproductive system problems. Respecting privacy is essential for building trust between a doctor and a patient and eliciting sensitive information about a patient's health. Most of the women refused to be examined by male students, even if chaperones were present.

The operating rooms were generally crowded. The doctors preferred us to observe the Caesarean sections from a distance and familiarize ourselves with the equipment (which included many speculums and suture materials). I was surprised to find that one of the surgeons trained at the same Kung Fu dojo as me. He reminded me that anyone can continue to pursue their hobbies, even someone as busy as a specialist surgeon. Seeing one C-section after another made us familiar with the procedure. We were instructed to watch and learn from a safe distance. But nothing can replace the thrill of wielding a scalpel and performing the operation. The heady smell of blood smoke became burned into our minds, whenever the doctors cauterized flesh.

The labor ward was a different story. The screams of pregnant mothers pierced the air. The nurses and doctors constantly ran from one patient to the next. It was a high-pressure, high-energy melting pot of patients, their families, and healthcare workers. My brother and I were teamed up with one of our other classmates. We were allocated to the labor ward for our night calls, which started at 4:00 pm and ended at 10:00 pm. Occasionally, if the supervising doctor allowed us and if the ward was quiet, we slipped out for a short while, to buy a meal from the nearby McDonald's, before being thrown back into the mix.

Some of my most memorable medical school experiences happened during the night calls. Usually, our team was the last to leave the obstetrics and gynecology department. We felt a sense of responsibility. We felt as if we were helping to make a difference in the lives of our patients. At night, there aren't many people who can cover for you. It's (more often than not) just you and the patient. That feeling of power can be intimidating but also motivating. Doctors are fond of reminding us that a day will come when we may need to manage a small clinic by ourselves. If that clinic is situated in a rural area, with limited resources; patient survival will largely depend on our clinical skills.

My time in the wards and the operating room exposed me to some ethically challenging situations. We witnessed many cases of abuse, sexual assault, and illegal (backstreet) abortions (which in many parts of my city are advertised illegally in public spaces). In South Africa, domestic violence and abuse of women and children is still a serious and persistent issue. Despite these significant social issues, during the gynecology rotation I witnessed, first-hand, the admirable strength and endurance of female patients and how they create new lives and support each other, even in the face of great suffering. These experiences compelled me to better understand motherhood.

ARCHAIC MATRIARCHY

A family of mongooses scurried away from me as I approached the weary edifice of Mahathma Gandhi Memorial Hospital and the gynecology ward: 7A. The words: "maternity ward entrance" were painted in cracked bold blue letters, above me.

Mongooses, much like humans, give birth to offspring, which are entirely dependent on parental support. Mother mongooses band together, much like the human mothers in ward 7A.

My colleagues and I were required to examine and observe patients in the antenatal clinic, gynecology ward, and the obstetrics theatre (where my clinical rotation began). The clinic and the ward were always busy, hot and crowded. The theatre (which had the only working air conditioner in the hospital) offered us relief from the summer heat.

Throughout those past three weeks, one thing became abundantly clear to me...the endurance of mothers is a force to behold.

Women's reproductive systems face an onslaught of stressors in the gynecology unit. Pipelles, punch biopsies, cone biopsies, and the intimidating weighted speculum (reminiscent of some ancient torture device) are just some of the terrifying tools that are used in gynecology. I observed a biopsy with my brother and one of our friendly senior doctors. A sharp instrument was used to cut out lesions in a woman's vagina. I had to help prepare the anesthetic (which numbs the pain). That still didn't stop me from wincing at the sight of the biopsy.

The ability of the ward 7A women to brave Pandora's box of gynecological conditions still astounds me.

The strength of women has been illustrated powerfully in legends of old. Consider the might of the Valkyries or the mythical Amazonian warriors who once battled the Ancient Greeks.

Carin Bondar, a mother, biologist, and the author of, "Wild Moms" analyzes motherhood and the nurturing of offspring, in different species. She notes some fascinating maternal behaviors in some of our more distant biological relatives, many of which resemble human motherly tendencies. Lion communes are a good example. Many lionesses have been known to form groups, to help nurse each other's cubs. I am reminded of this when I see the ward nurses teach mothers breastfeeding techniques.

Recapitulation theory, also known as, "ontogeny recapitulates phylogeny" states that the embryonic development of an individual organism (its ontogeny) follows the same path as the evolutionary history of its species. As we evolve, we supposedly resemble our genetic ancestors in some way e.g., the embryo of a pig or a fish can look similar to a human embryo at different stages of their respective developmental phases. This now-rejected idea has some truth to it, however. I feel that it is humbling to think that all living organisms are all inextricably linked and share some resemblance, no matter how small.

One of these similarities that we share...is the riskiness of childbirth.

Many animals risk their lives for their offspring. Cheetahs need to move their offspring frequently, to prevent predators from tracking them. Humans risk getting numerous infections and diseases during the birthing process.

The advent of modern medicine has helped us manage many of these diseases quite well. However, some problems have persisted. Many anthropologists claim that the painful birthing process is the product of an evolutionary compromise to accommodate walking in a species that also has an oversized brain-like humans. Groans of agony are not uncommon in the labor ward. Even from another side of the ward, I could recognize patients by their screams alone.

Enduring such pain (widely considered to be one of the worst kinds of pain that a human can experience), as well as an average of 9 months of pregnancy, is a testament to the investment that women will make to bring new life into the world.

Childbirth, in many cultures, is celebrated as a time of joy (one of our patients took a selfie with her newborn child, seconds after we watched her baby being delivered by Caesarean section). It was my first time seeing a C-section. I remember that moment vividly. It was my first day in the hospital theatre. The patient was conscious, while the doctors cut open her lower abdomen to remove her baby from her uterus. She felt no pain as an epidural anesthetic was given and was quite calm. A single green drape obscured her view of her internal organs, which were visible to me, the surgeons and the nurses. Her bright red blood was starkly juxtaposed against the green drapes and the cold metal instruments. I observed the clean incisions that the surgeon made with her scalpel. She cut quickly and deftly. It was clear that she had many years of experience doing C-sections. To my surprise, there was a lot of aggressive pulling involved. Sometimes, she needed the help of a theatre nurse to tear the tissue layers apart. It appeared to be a crude technique, but it was coordinated and effective. It was the first time that I realized how strong the uterus is. I was shocked to learn that a small organ of the reproductive system (approximately the size of a closed fist in non-pregnant women) can grow 500-1000 times its size, during pregnancy. It is incredibly well-designed. In textbooks, its shape resembles the skull of a bull, with two horns.

Then, we heard a cry...from a healthy baby girl. It was a shrill forced cry.

The nurse showed the baby to the mother, briefly. Tears of joy streamed from her eyes and she smiled in a way that I will not forget. During my years of clinical training, I have carefully observed how mothers smile when they see their first child for the first time. For many, it looks like a mix of shock, joy, and immense relief. I can only imagine how that feels: seeing another living organism that you created. It is a sudden, broad, welcoming smile that I imagine people make on a few, special occasions in their lives.

...but childbirth can be a time of great sorrow.

I witnessed the delivery of a dead fetus, during my gynecology rotation, for the first time as well.

It was a busy, humid night in the labor ward and most of us were sweating profusely. Flying ants were swarming outside the ward (as they usually do on humid South African summer nights). There was a lot of movement both outside and inside the hospital. Nurses and interns ran from patient to patient to help with deliveries. I was carefully taking blood from a pregnant woman when suddenly, a nurse called me over. She said that she needed me to help her fill in some forms for something urgent...

I arrived at the bedside at the exact moment that the nurse asked a mother to start bearing down to deliver a baby. The mother was a young Indian woman. She looked young (maybe 27 or 28). Beads of sweat dotted her forehead. Her expression was blank. The nurse was focused on delivering the baby, but she too was emotionless. Something felt unnerving...

No cry was heard, when the mother delivered.

The fetus, at first, looked alien and eerily still (I understood then, why the word, "stillbirth" seems so apt). It looked rubbery, with a dark maroon color, similar in appearance to coagulated blood. She asked if she could see the fetus. The nurse shifted hesitantly. "You might bond with the fetus" she warned. Nonetheless, the exhausted young mother gave a cursory glance at the organism that once developed within her…and stared listlessly at the ceiling. A sudden chill wind blew through the ward. Everything suddenly felt quiet, cold and still. The silence was deafening. I stood there, feeling helpless. I did not know if I could say anything that could help her. Her grief was palpable. It felt as if a great weight was suddenly placed on my shoulders.

The patient's partner beckoned to me and my colleague, a girl from my class, outside the patient's cubicle. We glanced at each other nervously, before stepping away from the patient's bed to join him. He assumed that I was one of the doctors. "She's been through too much" he said, with a look of desperation in his eyes. "Please don't let her take the stillbirth home. She'll grow attached to it and suffer more."

According to our ethics lectures, which are based mostly on South African laws, stillbirths are not classified as human and therefore are not afforded rights. A stillbirth is classified as pathological waste and is disposed of accordingly. All stillbirths must be registered and recorded by hospitals. I informed the patient's partner about this and clarified that I was just a medical student. The patient would not be allowed to take the stillbirth home with her. He nodded solemnly and continued to look anxiously at the ground with a pained expression on his face.

I could still feel the woman's sorrow. It was incredible how she felt such a deep connection with her unborn child. The nurse had seen many stillbirths before and approached the situation professionally. I did not know if that inured her to the pain of seeing someone lose their unborn child. Maybe it was a way for her to cope with seeing others endure great pain. I left the labor ward that night with a heavy heart and many questions. What could I have done to help? How did the patient feel? She never spoke a word to us.

Nature seems to have designed childbirth in such a way as to make it a harsh and unrelenting crucible, in keeping with the principles of natural selection. There was much blood, discharge, and screams of pain that echoed in my mind even as I walked through the hospital parking lot, in the gloaming, after patient intakes.

Despite this pain, motherhood, and childbirth remains a subject of beauty that has been immortalized in art. The many versions of Madonna and Child are evidence for the reverence of the motherly figure in society.

I think that as 4th-year medical students, we tend to place great emphasis on the clinical and objective aspects of childbirth. Maybe, we should also be more cognizant of its beauty and complexity. It is a source of immense joy and suffering.

Someday, we will be replaced. Every live birth and C-section I see now reminds me of transience. There is a Japanese term: "Mono no aware" which means: 'The awareness of the impermanence of things." I am only one of countless many who have followed the path of medicine. There will be countless others who will come after me. I have to do my best to facilitate their introduction into our world and help more women like the patient who lost her unborn child. I no longer wish to feel helpless in such a situation.

When we see childbirth, we witness a process that has created some of the most infinitely complex living organisms in existence, one that will continue ad infinitum...so long as we care for our mothers well.

7

ACUTE INTEGRATED CARE

Personal and social traumas

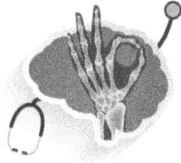

"Care shouldn't start in the emergency room."

— *JAMES DOUGLAS, LORD OF DOUGLAS*

S ome things in medicine are traumatizing. Get used to it! Aah! Integrated Acute Health, also known as the trauma block. Reviews about this clinical block, amongst my medical school friends, were mixed. Some of the students craved more clinical exposure. One of my friends even volunteered to work with an emergency team that rescued people from offshore oil rigs, which is incredibly cool. Some love the adrenaline rush of trauma and emergency medicine. Imagine broken limbs, snake bites, gunshot wounds and blood everywhere. This is the dream of every adrenaline junkie. Everything could be fine and then wham! Monitors start screaming in the ICU because a patient's oxygen levels are getting dangerously low. Our trauma block lasted 6 weeks and was mainly theoretical. The first 2 weeks were spent in the trauma department, which deals with fun things like stab wounds and gunshot injuries. Our trauma lectures were scheduled between 8:00 am and 12:00 pm, from Monday to Friday, at Albert Luthuli Hospital, the main quaternary hospital in our region. During the afternoons, we returned to our medical school skills labs, where we learned essential emergency medicine skills e.g., CPR and intubation. If a patient stopped breathing right in front of us, we needed to know what to do. The trauma lectures were fascinating, especially one presentation about treating snakebites and identifying common snakes in South Africa. A few students screamed when they saw the first PowerPoint slide...a collage of various deadly snakes. Some of them are commonly found in my province, such as the dreaded black mamba. Some of these snakes are 2-3m long and their venom could kill you in a few hours, if you don't get an antidote. Luckily, most of them are shy and avoid humans...

My following 2 weeks were spent in the Anaesthetics department of Prince Mshiyeni hospital, a 1200 bed regional hospital in Umlazi, one of the largest townships in South Africa. There is this stereotype that anesthesiologists are very laid-back. The hospital serves people from the surrounding area, up to and including parts of the Eastern Cape province. Understandably, patient caseloads were high there. But I had some good memories in that place.

Driving up to Prince Mshiyeni (which I called, "the hospital formerly known as Prince," as a joke) is a scene that I will not forget. The hospital's outer fences struggled to hold back the corrugated iron shacks that pushed against them. Chickens and wild dogs roamed freely outside the hospital. Despite many complaints from the hospital doctors about the limited resources; they worked effectively with what was available to them.

My memory of my first hospital intake at Prince Mshiyeni is still clear. Often the duration of intakes depends on how busy the hospital is. Some doctors work for 48 hours straight while on intake, in some of the busier South African hospitals. The atmosphere at Prince Mshiyeni changed slowly, but noticeably as day bled into night. Everything felt different in that hospital when night fell. The once bustling hallways became silent. Most of the patients were asleep. The dull lighting bathed the wards in a mysterious, somnolescent glow. The parking area and the surrounding settlements were pitch black. You could barely see beyond your hand. The experience was surreal.

I even befriended a few animals, during my intake nights, such as a litter of kittens, which found residence outside the wards, at night, and a chicken, which wandered into the intensive care unit (ICU) from a nearby informal settlement. We tried to chase it out...unsuccessfully. Nobody was bothered by the bird. It loved hanging around the resuscitation trolley for some reason. It eventually left the ICU after two days. I quipped that it was the worst case of chickenpox that I had ever seen. Coincidentally, my family ordered KFC that night...

We also spent some time working with an anesthetic simulator in Albert Luthuli hospital for a few days. The ongoing technological innovations at that hospital continue to impress me. There is a convincing replica of an operating theatre in the anesthetics department there. It had a resuscitation trolley, surgical equipment and everything! In the middle of the room was a humanoid dummy (which gave us all a feeling of uncanny valley). There were various tubes and ports inserted into the dummy's, "skin" to simulate a patient that had been prepared for theatre and was awaiting an anesthetic/analgesic drug. I volunteered to help with the demonstration. Interestingly enough, the head of the department was one of my uncle's friends, when he was in medical school. He asked me how I felt about the anesthetic block. I joked that people aren't supposed to feel anything when learning anesthetics. That one-liner works most of the time...

I injected an inducing agent (which helps the patient go to sleep) into one of the dummy's ports. It was amazing to see the dummy's breathing rate and heart rate slowly decrease. It felt almost like I was working with an actual patient.

Eventually, I did have the privilege of inducing an actual patient. I was supervised by an anesthesiologist who was fond of asking me to calculate patients' cerebral perfusion pressures (the amount of pressure needed to maintain blood flow to the brain). Some doctors love surprising us with questions, when we least expect it. When I started working with him, I watched him administer many epidural anesthetics (which involves injecting anesthetic into a space around the spinal cord to numb the lower body). I had seen the procedure a few times before during my gynecology block. We learned that choosing the appropriate anesthetic and analgesic drugs is a critical pre-operative step. Some patients can have life-threatening reactions to certain medications (e.g., malignant hyperthermia, which can present with symptoms like muscle rigidity and dangerously high body temperature >40 degrees C). When we started work in the orthopedics operating room, I was finally given the chance to administer one of the inducing agents myself. It was a milky white substance (in fact it looked exactly like condensed milk). I could feel a surge of power flowing through me. It was terrifying and galvanizing. I felt that I was actively helping the anesthetic team, but I was holding an incredibly dangerous drug in my hands. Some inducing agents are strictly regulated. Many of them are components of the lethal injection. Without proper supervision, it could be used to kill someone. Hypothetically, you could inject it into a random person on the street and you could kill them within a few minutes. The patient was then intubated by a flexible, slimy, jelly-like tube, to keep his airway open. The anesthesiologists monitored his heart rate and breathing closely.

1 week of our rotation was spent learning forensics-the application of science to criminal and civil laws-at Albert

Luthuli hospital. It was a brief, but fascinating exploration into the precise and calculated world of forensic medicine. Most of our time was spent attending lectures and workshops to help us identify common causes of death as well as how to determine if a person is dead (there have been rare reports of some patients being frozen alive in mortuaries). One of our tasks was to identify the contents of the sexual assault evidence kit. If a sexual assault victim came to us, we needed to know what to do. Learning the subject demands that you have good logical skills to piece together how a person died-just like Sherlock Holmes. You also need to know South African law very well (another example of how medicine has something to offer for everyone). Forensics may not be as glamorous as how CSI portrays it and you will probably do a lot more paperwork than you would imagine. In time, I befriended the heads of the forensics department. They told me that they came across many morbidly fascinating cases-including one instance of cannibalism, where the only collected evidence was a pot filled with maizemeal and a human leg. Most of your time will be spent around dead bodies. You might be recoiling in fear right now, but this subject does appeal to a niche group of people...

We spent the final 2 weeks of the block learning orthopedics. Many of my friends quipped that the orthopods (which are not to be confused with invertebrates with jointed appendages) resembled mechanics. Many of them seemed to have a very straightforward and hands-on approach to interacting with patients. Many orthopods are known as "ortho-bros": muscular, hands-on doctors who are strong enough to pick up patients. The discipline deals a lot with the muscles and bones of the body and requires doctors to have a great grasp of human anatomy. During our time in the department, we saw many broken bones and infected joints, especially in children (in fact, the Latin roots of the word: "orthopedics" mean: To straighten children-with reference to splinting their broken bones). Some of the equipment can be a bit intimidating (and subtlety resemble an iron maiden torture device) and include rods that are screwed into the bone. Just look up: "External fixation device" to see what I mean. It resembles a metal contraption from a Terminator movie.

There are many traumas that medical students experience. 6 years of our lives are spent earning our university degree. During this time, one experiences pain, which could be emotional, physical, psychological...the list goes on. Even though we are tasked with healing others; we must not forget our vulnerabilities.

During this block; I dealt with heartbreak. I could not help but compare my emotional trauma to the subjects that I was learning in the hospital at the time. Such moments have the potential to break us or strengthen us.

DIAGNOSING LOVE

The Sanskrit origin of the word, "love," lubhyati is also the root of the word, "desire." According to the Buddha: "Desire is the root of all suffering. I pondered this while studying a penetrating cardiac injury, during our trauma rotation at Inkosi Albert Luthuli Hospital. A hemorrhaged human heart was projected morbidly onto a lecture slide, at the front of our seminar room. It was the outcome of a rather unpleasant domestic dispute, involving a wife, her husband, and a kitchen knife. A prior discussion about the vicissitudes of breakups, with my colleagues at the hospital cafeteria, compelled me to ask this question..." How can such a powerful organ be hurt so intensely by teenage romance?"

Many dictionaries define beauty as a combination of qualities that please the aesthetic senses, especially the sight. Other scientists associate beauty with a number: 1.618.

This number, the gloriously named, "Golden Ratio," is a product of the Fibonacci sequence, which is formed by adding one number to the number that precedes it. Many studies have found this supposedly divine number to be important in determining many aspects of human biology: the structure of DNA, the branching of coronary arteries...and the dimensions of the face...a part of our anatomy that is a central feature of aesthetic beauty, as well as a converging point for sensory information. Some studies suggest that people are perceived to be more beautiful if their facial anatomy follows this ratio. (I don't actively encourage other medical students to measure their patients' faces, to confirm this).

Now, imagine this: You're sitting in your medical school or hospital cafeteria when suddenly, an attractive colleague walks toward you. First, something dilates...your pupils (I don't know what you were thinking). Your autonomic nervous system is kicked into overdrive, as your body unleashes a primordial biological and physiological maelstrom designed to propagate the human race. Your cortisol levels increase (a stress hormone that is important for your fight-or-flight response). Your vagus nerve stimulates your gastrointestinal tract. You prepare to say something and prove your genetic suitability as a mate...until you realize that she was just walking towards the pathology lab to deliver a blood sample (not towards you); she is 29 (which means that you are too young for her) and she is wearing an engagement ring.

...What just happened?

According to Seshadri KG in his 2016 article for the journal of endocrinology and metabolism...you experienced lust, one of the three intertwined components of love.

An infinitude of literature and songs about this phenomenon, love, exists. Humans have attempted to comprehend it for millennia (think of the Song of Songs from the Bible's Old

Testament...or the hit single by the Kpop group, Twice, "What is love?" As Lurr, from the brilliant TV series, Futurama roared so aptly: "this concept of, wuv confuses and infuriates us!"

Seshadri KG states:" Love may be defined as an emergent property of an ancient cocktail of neuropeptides and neurotransmitters."

Consider this scenario: You end up dating the colleague with a golden ratio face. She happens to be fond of younger men; was only wearing a "friendship ring" and she loves video games... (a man can dream). You both then have a few amorous rendezvous in and around Durban. You enjoy long walks along the beach. You dine together and eventually; you grow attached to her. It feels fantastic! It's as if you are floating on air. De Boer et. al identified hormones like oxytocin (the trust hormone), vasopressin, dopamine, and their receptors as crucial players in the romantic orchestra that galvanizes the body's desire for social bonding (which becomes ever more important, when one returns home, fatigued after a long night hospital call, and in need of companionship). There is also evidence for a role of other chemical signals like serotonin, cortisol, nerve growth factor, and testosterone in love and attachment.

Dario Maestripieri of Psychology Today describes this beautiful physiological tempest as the source of much of human motivation. He believes that sexual desire is essential to motivate humans to mate, raise children and propagate our lineage. However, romantic love and pair-bonding developed as a result of infants, becoming needier. As their brains grew, their development required more time and they were thus vulnerable for longer. The father's involvement and bi-parental care became necessary. Natural selection had to come up with a way to motivate men and women to stay together for as long as it took to raise a child successfully. Romantic love seemed to be a logical solution.

And naturally, your body rewards you for falling in love. Multiple studies seem to confirm this. You live longer; your immunity improves and blood flow to the skin…and other areas, increases. I have joked that many doctors should write, "fall in love" as part of their management plan for many patients. If love is a drug…can our medical aids not cover it? Is it technically possible to prescribe it?

The chemist, Paracelsus, the father of toxicology, is credited for creating the classical toxicology maxim:" All things are poison, and nothing is without poison, the dosage alone makes it so a thing is not a poison." If we define love as a drug (a medicine or other substance that has a physiological effect when ingested or otherwise introduced into the body) then love can also have a poisonous dose…

Love, like many drugs, is deadly, when the administered dose is too small (loneliness or neglect), if it is suddenly withdrawn (heartbreak) or if the dose becomes uncontrollably high (jealousy and obsession).

Often, many victims of heartbreak describe the sensation of losing a loved one as physical pain: "It feels like being stabbed by a hot knife" or, "I felt like I was slapped in the face. "There is a disease named after heartbreak…heartbreak syndrome. The Japanese refer to it as takotsubo cardiomyopathy, a rare pathology, categorized by catecholamine mediated stunning of the heart. The condition is named after Japanese pots, that are used to trap octopi (the apex of the heart resembles the shape of this pot, in patients with this disease). Patient's (usually the elderly) are at risk of suffering from this disease after losing someone about whom they cared deeply. This disease is also surprisingly prevalent in communities, which practice voodoo magic. Those who strongly believe that they are cursed by voodoo magic, tend to experience autonomic nervous system dysfunction as a result of feelings of overwhelming hopelessness.

Those who are heartbroken experience similar feelings of hopelessness.

A 2016 Maryland study identified three main heartbreak coping strategies in a group of forlorn participants: Reappraisal, distraction, and situation selection (e.g., avoiding gifts/cues that were received from an ex). The study also suggests that love can be controlled through various behavioral and cognitive strategies (the so-called: "up-regulation and down-regulation" of love). The idea that love can be controlled is compelling and begs the question: "How do medical students manage heartbreak, in our demanding careers?" We may wonder how many of our students and consultants manage to force themselves to work, despite carrying a heavy heart. How does a doctor work effectively, after suffering from heartbreak or the loss of a loved one? Does heartbreak delay recovery periods, in patients? Should heartbreak be classified as a disease that warrants sick leave, as a result of all of the strain that it places on the human body? Relationships (both romantic and platonic) are important determinants of health for everyone, including healthcare professionals. I have known many doctors who soldier on each day, even after suffering great heartbreak. They can get frustrated and feel overwhelmed. It takes a toll on them. Sometimes, talking to them and taking the time to listen can make a world of difference. A surgeon at Prince Mshiyeni opened up to me, after we chatted about life in the operating room. He told me that he lost his wife. His work numbed his pain and gave him purpose.

We may try to dissect love, and analyze it clinically. However, those who have experienced love for another will know that love is anything but clinical. It can feel like a panacea as well as a disease, in different situations. It is the stimulus that triggers a torrent of emotions, within us, as well as discord between our minds and hearts. As a medical student, love (of our work, our family, or another) is what keeps us going during the long nights and the 24-hour work shifts. The biological heart, the core of our bodies, gives us the blood we need to save patients and survive. The metaphorical heart, the center of our souls, gives us a reason to do it.

The trauma wards and the emergency rooms lay bare the vulnerability of humans. In the past few years of my clinical training, I have seen numerous cases of stabbed lungs and hearts; gunshot wounds, and blunt injuries (many caused by airborne beer bottles). The human body hangs in a constant delicate balance, known as homeostasis. If you lose too much blood, you could die. The solution is then to replace the lost blood. If you cannot breathe properly, you could die. The solution is then to find out why the person cannot breathe: Is it a problem with the airways or is the blood not carrying enough oxygen? You then address those problems, sequentially, using evidence that you collected by asking the patient questions (if they are conscious), examining them, and doing other necessary investigations (such as bedside tests, laboratory tests, and imaging tests e.g., X-rays). Medicine requires logic. This applies to all medical disciplines.

There is a large public hospital known as King Edward hospital, which is situated right next to our campus. Like most hospitals in Durban, it has seen better days. Parts of the ceiling are exposed, such that you can see the pipelines and coils of electrical wire that crisscross through the hospital, like an aged infected vascular system. The staff there do their best with the available resources. My colleagues and I were required to spend one night intake in the emergency room there.

Initially, everything was quiet. It was a rectangular room, filled with patient beds, monitors, and desks for completing administrative work. There were two patients with fractured limbs who were stable. Around 8:00 pm there was a sudden influx of patients. There was only one available doctor on call for the night. He asked my brother and me to wheel one of the patients with a fractured leg to the nearby X-ray room, as soon as her condition stabilized. I have had some fun encounters with radiologists. Some of them love to grill students and doctors for making X-ray requests, like an academic kangaroo court. It can be nerve-wracking, but you have to stand your ground and support your reasoning. Many of them ask for thorough explanations for why you are asking for X-rays or other imaging studies like CT scans. You'll be lucky if you get your patients' CT scans or MRI scans on time, in a public hospital. The queue for those investigations is usually very long. It is good to stay in the radiologists' good books if you want to get imaging study results for your patients on time. Luckily, the radiologist liked us, so she accepted our patient, with a smile. Charm, kindness, and good manners go a long way in hospitals.

We rushed back to the emergency room in time to take a history from an adolescent patient who was whipped multiple times by a sjambok (a long whip used for herding cattle, that can also double as a weapon for self-defense). His back was marked by multiple long, deep cuts. His blood was a bright scarlet color. He cried in pain as he clenched his pillow. This is not an uncommon site in South African emergency rooms. We learned from our pathology lectures that severe muscle damage can result in renal failure in some patients (these are called crush injuries). His mother was hysterical, but we calmed her down by explaining that he could be treated for his condition and there was a good chance that there would be no long-term complications. We reported our findings to the doctor on call, who continued management for the patient. After a short while, he examined a few X-rays with us. By then, it was a little after 9:45 pm and he advised that we should return home. We asked if he needed any extra help. He sighed and told us that he could handle things just fine. The bags under his eyes were deep and dark. He signed our logbooks and returned to face the growing wave of new patients.

Health workers are not invincible. We endure the same traumas as everyone else-both physical and emotional. The human heart, despite its incredible complexity, can be devastated by a stab wound or a stress response caused by heartbreak.

We face multiple stressors in the form of long working hours, personal issues, patient deaths, which can all contribute to physician burnout. Much like trauma management, the management of these traumatizing stressors is logical, with a strong focus on maintaining homeostasis. If you feel burnt out, find out the reason why and seek help as soon as you can. If you feel like you're not getting enough sleep, find out why and adjust your schedule. This is of course easier said than done. Seek help if you find it hard to identify what could be causing you to suffer.

My family helped me through my heartbreak-which is just another trial that we face in medical school and life. People have a misconception that all healthcare professionals are revered diagnostic wizards with all the answers to our problems. There are times when we get hurt. There are needlestick injury protocols in almost every hospital in my province. Doctors make mistakes. Because of the HIV epidemic in South Africa, even a poke from a small needle could put you at risk of getting HIV, if you used that needle on a patient. We are constantly reminded to watch our needles, never recap them and dispose of them in sharps containers. Despite this, many healthcare professionals suffer from needlestick injuries and other diseases. One of my colleagues, a healthy adolescent, suffered from TB symptoms in his first year of internship.

Trauma, like many aspects of healthcare, is closely linked to social determinants of health. Many of the trauma cases that we have seen are related to preventable causes such as stab wounds, gunshots, and motor vehicle collisions. For our public health selectives project, we researched motor vehicle collisions in Durban during our 2nd to 4th year of medical school to try to evaluate pedestrian knowledge of road safety, in our city. We then created a workshop with a few community members to spread awareness of safer road-crossing behavior. In my 5th year of medical school, I started presenting for a TV show. In one episode, I interviewed our provincial spokesperson for the South African Police Services, to identify measures that they instituted to reduce violent crimes, during the holiday season. I even had a chance to speak directly to victims of violent crimes and people who lost family members to incidents such as hijackings and assault. The responses were often very similar. They all reported that they felt devastated and in need of justice. These were ordinary people, whose lives were completely changed by crime. Hearing their stories was a jarring reminder that we need to solve major societal problems if we want to see healthcare in South Africa drastically improve. During my 5th year of medical school, on one night, Chris Hani Baragwanath Hospital (the third largest hospital in the world at the time) reported an empty emergency room for the first time in history, since its opening in the early 1900s. For the first time, there were no patients admitted for stabbings or gunshot wounds. To put things in perspective, emergency room admissions account for 70% of all of the hospital's patient admissions. This only happened after alcohol sales were banned, during the COVID-19 global pandemic. A notable fall in cases of motor vehicle collisions and violence were recorded as well. Addressing social issues results in palpable changes in healthcare.

It is very easy to feel cloistered in medical school. Many students will go to campus or hospital, attend lectures, acquire signatures for our logbooks and then go home. It is easy to follow this flow. I can understand this. Many students feel tired, hungry, and overworked in medical school and often do not feel the need to do anything more than the bare minimum that is required to pass our modules, at the end of a long day. This behavior then persists in internship and beyond. Many of my friends who are doing their internships then report that work in hospitals feels like a Red Queen Effect-we are constantly pushing ourselves to stay in the same place. Every day, we see the same cases-gunshot wounds, stabbed lungs, and wonder: "When will it end?" We do our part by addressing the downstream problems. We drain the blood and air out of the chest cavity. But, the most effective long-term solution is to address the upstream causes of the stab wounds. We must stop people from getting stabbed in the first place. We must teach people that violence is not the answer. We must speak out against injustices like sexual abuse and drunk driving. Education is a powerful tool. I have seen the good that can arise when a nation is united against a common problem. When the COVID-19 pandemic affected the world in 2020, thousands of South Africans encouraged others to wear masks to help slow down the spread of the novel coronavirus. We also spoke out against gender-based violence that festered during our national lockdown. The president at the time, Cyril Ramaphosa, even directly addressed the public on these matters through a series of state of the nation addresses. It was a powerful step in the right direction that motivated others to condemn a social ill e.g., through social media. Changing societal mindsets requires a combined effort.

Everyone, the president, you, me, we all need to do our part. It is not only the responsibility of the government and the healthcare system. If we work together, we can help everyone. We will see fewer cases of stabbings, gunshot wounds, gender-based violence…and hopefully ease the burden for those doctors and other members of society who are dealing with personal traumas.

8

PRIMARY HEALTH CARE

Upstream solutions

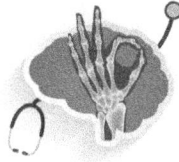

"I loved clinical practice, but in public health, you can impact more than one person at a time. The whole society is your patient."

— *TOM FRIEDEN*

Primary healthcare is where we learn the bread and butter of clinic work. It is where we learn skills that help us treat any common condition that a patient can present with at a grassroots level. If a patient comes to us with pneumonia, we can handle it. If a patient has a heart attack, we can bust out the necessary medication. So, what is primary healthcare? Simply put, Primary healthcare focuses on the health of individuals, communities, and families by considering their needs and preferences, addressing broader determinants of health (e.g., access to water or shelter and socioeconomic factors), and emphasizing physical, mental, and social health and wellbeing. We look at the patient holistically and we assess his/her situation.

My first exposure to community health was the, "Making a Difference Project" (during our 1st year of medical school) and the "Selectives program" (which we worked on, from year 2 to year 4 of medical school).

The, "Making a Difference project" was part of our curriculum and demanded us to do exactly what its name suggests...to make a difference-a positive change (preferably in our community). Firstly, we were assorted into random groups (of 3-4 people). We chose to make a difference in a small church near our medical school. We saw the church services as an opportunity to educate community members about the importance of hygiene (through effective hand washing techniques), nutrition, and HIV/AIDS prevention (e.g., safer sexual practices and the importance of condom use).

The "Selectives program" taught me some important lessons about community-oriented primary health care and becoming a so-called, "agent of change" in my community (our public health lecturers love this term). For me, this term is associated with someone who can significantly change a community for the better, in some way.

During my 3 years of working on our Selectives project, with my twin brother and another colleague; I had many fascinating opportunities to meet patients and their families, within their communities (e.g., home visits). During our public health and family medicine lectures, I learned to integrate the theory of these two disciplines of health into my interaction with patients and their families. COPC (Community-oriented primary care) is a system that combines all these principles: epidemiology (studies of patterns and distributions of disease), primary care, preventive medicine, and health promotion into an effective systematic approach to healthcare. This creates what is known as the COPC cycle, which requires a community diagnosis to be made and prioritized, for a detailed problem assessment of a community to be made. We then plan an intervention. The intervention is then implemented, evaluated, reassessed, and prioritized again, thus completing the COPC cycle. Put simply…1. We find a problem in a community. 2. We plan ways to solve it. 3. We implement an intervention to solve the problem. 4. We see if the intervention was worthwhile, and we change it if necessary. I have learned that COPC is a continuous process that is intended to meet the health needs of a defined population, through planned integration of public health with primary care practice. This is a big task. It is not easy to change the way things are, but one person can make a difference.

Being connected to the community in which we work as healthcare professionals is incredibly important. For me, it was also a great way to make new friends. For example, one of our assignments as part of the Selectives project was to visit the home of a patient who had a chronic illness. To maintain patient confidentiality, I will not reveal any personal details. We will call him Mr. Patrick (not his real name).

Mr. Patrick has chronic high blood pressure and bronchitis (inflammation of the airways which is associated with excess mucus buildup and can cause difficulty breathing). His cough used to get really bad during winter. He still visits his local clinic, to collect his medication. He now smokes and drinks more frequently than before. He also understands that his persistent smoking is the reason why his chronic bronchitis has worsened. He does not feel that his inhaler or other medications are helping him. He is still willing to change his habits, but he feels that it is very difficult, since he has smoked and consumed alcohol for many years. Discouraging patients from smoking is still a big challenge for us. The patient also has a newfound desire for female companionship and feels that the comfort of a girlfriend might help, "stabilize" him, emotionally. Mr. Patrick revealed fears about aging and illness, discord within his family as well as concerns about stress coping mechanisms. You can understand what I mean when I said that we get to know patients very personally. We ask them questions that they never asked themselves such as:" What kind of toilet do you use?"

Calling Mr. Patrick to arrange my final home visit with him felt bittersweet. Learning intimate knowledge about his biomedical and social history as well as his ideas, concerns, fears, expectations, and emotions allowed me to develop a great deal of empathy and compassion for him and his family. I arranged an afternoon visit with Mr. Patrick when he finished work. He seemed sorrowful to hear that it was my final home visit. When somebody trusts you with so much of his/her personal information, it feels natural to develop a friendship.

Patient interaction at many of the public hospitals that I visited during my 3rd and 4th years of medical school were rushed, usually because of excessive patient caseloads. This means that there isn't always enough time to get to know all your patients very well. My home visits allowed me enough time to gain a thorough holistic view of a patient's clinical as well as social and contextual situation. I had to learn almost everything about him (even how he disposes of his rubbish). Mr. Patrick explained to me that discussing illness and health with somebody else greatly relieved him of his stress and latent fears about disease and aging. I have seen, first-hand that the patient-doctor interaction demands compassion and empathy, in conjunction with clinical proficiency, for care to be effective. The patient may grow to trust your clinical decision, if they see that you actively care for them as a person. They can tell if you see them as a person instead of, "just another patient". It's a 6th sense that patients have.

The home visit was a poignant experience for me. It is uncommon for people to willingly allow you to enter their personal space and reveal their vulnerabilities to you. I have come to realize that medicine does not just belong in healthcare facilities. Healthcare affects everyone. Sometimes, just visiting a friend and talking to them can be an effective form of therapy. Listening to them, showing that you care, and expressing a clear interest in their personal and social wellbeing can go a long way. Now and then I still hear from Mr. Patrick. The selectives experience afforded me many fascinating encounters with patients, such as a discussion with a 65-year-old stroke patient, who asked me to simply explain how a stroke can cause walking difficulties; or a chance to bandage a young woman's trauma wound. These are but a few of the many experiences that have allowed me to develop empathy and compassion for my future patients. I now appreciate each new patient-doctor interaction as an opportunity to develop meaningful professional intimacy.

Visiting primary health care facilities, such as clinics, during the selectives project also allowed me opportunities to meet many other health care practitioners, within my immediate community (mostly GPs), which improved my abilities to collaborate with other key contributors to the health and wellbeing of my community. We are all a team. We should never feel that we are isolated or that we should shoulder the burden of the entire healthcare system. At one of the clinics, our selectives group spearheaded road safety prevention programs and managed clinic resources, with the clinic nurses. This helped me become a better health manager and leader. We increased our number of health promotion opportunities by encouraging safer pedestrian behaviors amongst patients, at every consultation, which helped us further develop our health advocacy skills.

During the project; we were required to keep a journal of our thoughts (about life in the clinics and patient-doctor interactions). As a result of my reflective writing practice; I developed a deep appreciation for medical writing (which also helped me write this book). In the future, I intend to continue writing about my experiences with patients and our local community, to remind others about the importance of appreciating the small things, during patient interactions. This can be a sigh of relief or something barely noticeable like the tensing of muscles when a person hears bad news. Writing is one of my more therapeutic pastimes. The new research skills that I acquired during the selectives program encouraged me to pursue novel areas of research and health promotion in other disciplines, like genetics. To be selective, by definition, is to choose the most suitable or best qualified of something. The selectives program required me to choose/select key public health skills that interested me (health advocacy and health promotion), study them, and practice them.

During my 4th year of medical school; I was allocated to a small and busy clinic in Phoenix, for our family medicine block. I remember my first day there, well. My twin brother was assigned to the same clinic as me. We make a great team. It was good to have the extra company. The winding roads to the clinic were dusty and the sun's heat was relentless. We were in a hurry to find our supervising doctor, who was supposed to give us our orientation at the clinic.

Phoenix primary healthcare clinic is constantly teeming with patients. It feels like a small slice of India: hot and constantly bustling with people from all walks of life. My first impression of the clinic was one of…admiration. Every day, a small team of doctors and nurses brace themselves and guide seemingly overwhelming waves of new patients into the different clinic compartments, where they are examined and management plans are prepared for them.

Most of the patients were affected by hypertension (high blood pressure) and/or diabetes. Many elderly Indian men and women presented with eye and kidney pathology there. They frequented the clinic to receive their routine blood pressure monitoring and blood tests.

During my second week in the clinic; I walked by a long queue of women awaiting routine pap smears before I arrived at one of the doctor's consulting rooms. I met a friendly registrar from the University of Cape Town (UCT) there. Students from UKZN and UCT share a fun rivalry. We tell people that our clinical skills are better. They tell people that their theoretical knowledge is better. The registrar instructed me to clerk a middle-aged Indian boilermaker, who was suffering from chronic hypertension, chronic cough, and persistent lower back pain.

"Boilermaker?" I thought. My first thought was possible lung pathology (a connection that was taught to us during our 2nd-year anatomical pathology lectures). History taking (using the reliable Calgary Cambridge guide-which is taught to first-year medical students at our university) revealed tell-tale signs of chronic obstructive pulmonary disease (or COPD-a a chronic inflammatory lung disease that causes obstructed airflow from the lungs). Clinical examination revealed little besides a raised blood pressure, a mild cough and mild diffuse wheezes (which have a musical sound). Those signs could have been easily missed if the clinic background noise was slightly louder.

"Is there anything else that you wish to discuss with me?" I asked my patient casually (nearing the end of the examination). "Well, my wife of 41 years deceived me and now I'm preparing for a divorce," he said…as a matter-of-fact, throw-away remark.

"…I'm sorry to hear that" I muttered. My patient had waited until the end of the examination to share such a valuable part of his social history. The patient expected treatment for his respiratory pathology and not his social pathology. I wondered if this experience reflected the purely biomedical and clinical approach to patient wellbeing that has become commonplace in hospitals and clinics, that are bombarded with overwhelming patient case-loads. We sometimes become so focused on treating the disease, that we forget that we must treat the person with the disease. Some patients only expect us to manage their disease and not their social problems, which often contribute largely to their diseases (e.g., smoking, alcoholism, divorce…). At first, I was not sure how much I could do, besides sympathize with the patient and attempt to empathize with him. I also referred the patient to the social worker at the clinic. The patient revealed that he found solace amongst his fellow churchgoers. They aided him throughout his journey of emotional recovery.

I joined a few short consultations with two other interns. I quietly noted the average consultation time: 5 minutes, which is hardly enough time to take a full history (including a social history) from each of the 40+ patients who are seen by the interns daily. I needed to create a more concise abridged version of my history taking question list to ensure that pertinent patient social history details were not missed. Taking a patient history does not mean sticking to a rigid checklist. Every patient is different and we must adapt our questioning styles accordingly. Some patients are quiet and offer one-word answers. Others love to talk and you have to shorten your own answers to ensure that you finish the consultation on time.

I was initially unaware of the available social service facilities at the clinic. After asking a few nurses and navigating my way through the labyrinth of patients and interleading cubicles; I eventually found the social services worker. She was eager to discuss the numerous social issues that encumber most of the clinic patients. Divorce and domestic abuse are just a few of the common problems. My conversation with her reinforced my desire to better understand the social context of the clinic patients as well as the cultural context in which social issues arise. Perhaps then, I could better empathize with my patients and suggest more culturally appropriate ways for my patients to manage their social problems. It helps to know where your patients come from.

In another incident, a middle-aged Indian woman barged into one of the consultation rooms, while my brother and I were clerking a patient with hypertension. In a desperate attempt to skip the queue, she bombarded us with her list of symptoms: chronic pain, incontinence, blurred vision...while the other patient and I watched her, mildly perplexed. She proudly exclaimed that she was diagnosed with Sjogren's syndrome (an autoimmune disorder characterized by dry eyes and dry mouth) and acute renal azotemia (elevated levels of urea and other nitrogen compounds in the blood, as a result of kidney disease). She must have assumed that people with rarer diseases would receive more attention than people with more common pathologies. An intern quietly ushered her out of the room. I could not help but wonder (while still processing the patient's rant) how patients were triaged in the clinic and how the long waiting hours in the queue disrupted their daily activities. It is sometimes easy to forget these small details when you are swamped by patients. It is easy to become desensitized to the way things are.

During our time in the Phoenix clinic; we befriended many doctors, dental surgeons, and a dedicated ophthalmic nurse. They were all very welcoming and enjoyed our company. One of our assignments for our family medicine block was to complete, "a bingo card." We needed to familiarize ourselves with the other ancillary services and departments that helped the clinic operate smoothly (e.g., waste disposal, HIV/AIDS counseling services, and social services). We were tasked with collecting signatures from workers in these departments, which we then marked off in our logbooks. We even visited the clinic pharmacy, which was much bigger than I initially expected. Usually, we see the small windows, where patients collect their medications. After navigating our way through the convoluted passages of the clinic, we found out what was happening behind those windows. It was a huge operation with rooms filled with boxes of medication, packaging equipment, students, pharmacists in white lab coats, and administrative staff. It was a great opportunity to learn about the inner workings of a primary healthcare clinic and identify areas, where improvements could be made. It takes a huge amount of manpower to operate a clinic smoothly. A lot of it happens in the background. At the pharmacy, my group at the clinic discovered that antibiotics were occasionally being administered to patients with the flu. Antibiotics are often ineffective in patients with the flu and contribute to antibiotic resistance in patients (which means that some antibiotics can become less effective). It is a serious global problem.

A conversation with the social worker allowed me a chance to better understand the referral pathway for sexual assault patients (to Mahathma Gandhi Memorial Hospital), where the sexual assault and evidence collection kits are available. The infection control manager taught us the differences between the red and green disinfectants that are ubiquitous in most South African healthcare facilities. The green disinfectant contains an emollient, which should be used for cleaning the hands (not the red disinfectant). It is easy to forget that so many people work in the background, like cogs in a giant machine, to make our healthcare system operate.

Meeting the eye clinic nurse at Phoenix Primary Healthcare Centre offered me great insight into the diversity of nursing specialties. I learned that ophthalmic nurses play an extremely useful role in terms of identifying, assessing, and managing patients with a variety of common eye diseases e.g., blindness, cataracts, myopia (short-sightedness), hypermetropia (far-sightedness), scratched corneas, and eye trauma. A stabbed eye is not a pleasant sight.

I also learned about the methods of testing for visual acuity in illiterate patients as well as quick and effective techniques for calming a child, before assessing his/her eyes. Placing the child on his/her mother's lap and distracting him/her with a colorful toy really helps. Toys are very useful when working with children. The ophthalmic nurse also played a great role in adjusting and updating eye health policies at the clinic (e.g., preparing budgets for financial officers at the clinic). She also advocated for free spectacles for children and elderly patients, who were diagnosed with eye pathologies. She also referred eye clinic patients with possible complications to McCord's hospital-one of our main local hospitals for patients with eye pathologies. Her dedication to community service was admirable. Thanks to her, I have a better understanding of the conditions that can be managed at the clinic versus conditions that require referral. The referral pathway is essentially a guide that tells us where to send patients who have certain conditions. If we can't treat them at the clinic, then it may be best to refer them to a hospital. In Phoenix, eye problems related to diabetes and high blood pressure were the most common conditions that we saw during our time in the eye clinic. These diseases are generally common amongst Indians in Durban.

Overall, my experiences at the eye clinic were interesting and have deepened my appreciation for the services of ophthalmic nurses as well as the diversity of the entire healthcare multidisciplinary team. Health facilities work like a syncytium. We're cells in one giant body. Everyone plays their part. Security guards, dentists, cleaners, doctors, specialists are but a few of the many team members who make our health system work. My brother and I were fond of walking past the dental department, which was run by a group of welcoming Indian doctors and nurses. In Indian culture, it is common knowledge that Indian aunties and mothers love to feed people. If you visit an Indian home, there is a good chance that an Indian aunty will keep filling up your plate, even if you protest and say that you are full. Whenever the dental team brought some extra curry or biryani to work (a delicious Indian dish made with seasoned rice and meat, fish, or vegetables) they shared it with us. My brother and I thanked them at the end of our rotation, by buying them a chocolate cake. I was amazed by the strong sense of community in the clinic.

Developing close and intimate relationships with the community members was important to elicit important, private information about their chronic diseases. It is an integral part of caring for patients. It was apparent that chronic conditions (such as diabetes and hypertension) were common problems in the Phoenix community. This is multifactorial and again is closely linked to social determinants of health (e.g., diet, culture and exercise), Many of these diseases follow certain patterns that can be predicted. During my family medicine block, I was also participating in an online science communication course that was offered by Stellenbosch University. For our final course assignment; I wrote an essay about the possibility of using artificial intelligence to help doctors manage patients with certain predictable disease patterns, in a setting such as the Phoenix clinic. However, I emphasized that human care and patient-doctor interaction will always have a place in the medical field. During my 4th year of medical school; the use of artificial intelligence in medicine was rapidly gaining interest. I submitted my essay to Nature for a writing competition and was fortunate to have my article ranked in the top 10% of submissions. It was an honor to see that my experiences in a small clinic in Phoenix were gaining the interest of some prominent science writers. It certainly encouraged me to refine my writing and reflect on my interactions with patients more often.

MBCHB AND AI

Quickly recognizing a patient's condition can feel like a flash of intuitive lightning. At least that is how I felt when I correctly diagnosed someone with DiGeorge Syndrome: A condition that can cause recurrent infections in patients. The patient, from Addington hospital, in Durban, boasted a treasure trove of clinical signs. Hunting for every clue and piecing them together to solve a clinical conundrum is the raison d'être for the aspiring diagnostic wizard...but, as humans, we still make mistakes.

During the first four years of my medical training, I learned that the art of diagnosing patients is based on patterns, which are identified through rigorous history taking, clinical examination, and investigations. Consider Tuberculosis and HIV, a sinister duo that, together, infect thousands of new South Africans, annually. Consequently, Durban's hospital wards have become a cruel democracy of appearance: Wasting, night sweats, fever, chronic cough...the list goes on. These are common symptoms in patients who have HIV and TB.

What if some device could identify these common patterns as well as suggest appropriate treatment regimens? Imagine if a machine could ebb the daily torrent of patients at our public hospitals. Could robotic efficiency eliminate human error: a common cause of misdiagnosis and over-prescription of medication?

Enter the A.I. doctor.

Artificial intelligence (A.I.) is a groundbreaking way to train computer systems such that they can execute tasks that would normally be done by intelligent organisms. These computers discover, reason, and learn, much like my fellow medical students. These machines learn through symbols and the formation of complex arborizing networks, that mimic the connections of the neurons that we see in our physiology textbooks.

My hospital and clinic rotations, within KwaZulu Natal, as well as my epidemiology lecturers, have taught me that HIV, TB, hypertension, and diabetes mellitus are some of the most common diseases that plague patients in our province. At the Primary Health Care Centre in the Phoenix community, this deadly quartet is quotidian. Hundreds of work hours are spent performing repetitive tasks: History taking, HIV testing and taking blood ad infinitum. We identify these diseases because of consistent pathological patterns and treat these patients robotically according to management algorithms. Surely, an actual robot...an AI doctor would be perfect for this task?

AI machines in healthcare already excel at these errands. My undergraduate colleagues can attest to the benefits of using ECG machines, which suggest possible diagnoses for patients' heart conditions.

Many of these machines even surpass the abilities of expert consultants. AI machines trained to identify common skin cancers can diagnose more accurately than expert dermatologists. This has profound potential for resource-limited areas in South Africa (especially in rural areas) as well as the rest of the world. A dearth of available trained medical staff is already noticeable in wealthier provinces, such as Gauteng, where the population continues to increase, without a corresponding increase in health staff. There are many reasons for this, including a limited budget for remunerating skilled healthcare professionals. One must also account for the South African brain drain and the preference for doctors to live and work in urban areas. A Harvard business review by Brian Kalis predicted that the top 10 AI applications that could change healthcare will include machines that serve as virtual nursing assistants as well as administrative workflow assistants (to help doctors manage documentation more efficiently). These workflow assistants could also reduce the risk of burnout in healthcare workers, which is a serious problem. The use of these machines as AI doctors for making preliminary diagnoses could also save millions of Rands for the South African healthcare system, which like Atlas, wearily carries an immense weight: the weight of our nation's wellbeing.

It is not uncommon in Durban hospitals or clinics to find only 5 doctors per department (if you are lucky), attending to 60 or more patients, per day. I saw this in Prince Mshiyeni and the clinic in Phoenix. These doctors are often too busy to help students' attempts at diagnosing patients. Imagine an AI doctor that is readily available at any time of the day to receive patient data for common conditions; diagnose patients more accurately than a human consultant and suggest management plans. These machines don't have families to go back home to and are not limited by the need to sleep or eat, after a 20-hour work shift. AI doctors could be saviors in understaffed healthcare centers... and they would not berate us like the more irritable consultants. It is a dream that I hope will be realized in our lifetime.

Is the AI doctor the panacea for our healthcare problems? No.

"Why do I have cervical cancer, doctor?" (Patients tend to call us doctors, even though we are still undergraduates). This was a question I was asked by a young aspiring film star, in the gynecology ward of a hospital in Phoenix. She nicknamed my brother," Stones" because his palpating hands are strong. The desperate look in her eyes was piercing. I placed my arm on her shoulder and told her, "We will find out and we will do our best to help you, Ms."

A machine cannot do this as well as a human. An AI doctor could have diagnosed her. But it could not comfort her or answer her all-important question, "Why?" That is where we humans come in.

Diagnosis in Greek means to, "know apart." Effective and innovative healthcare demands that we know together and learn together, as man and machine, MBCHB and AI, skilled diagnosis, and skilled care. Imagine the power of our chimeric abilities, if we had affordable AI doctors in every clinic. Patients could be diagnosed before we even see them, which gives us more time to care for them.

When I wrote this article, I was prompted to think about the importance of staying up-to-date with new medical innovations and technology, in our discipline. The first 3 years of our medical school degree were dedicated to forming a strong foundation for understanding medical science.

We did not have much time in the laboratory, but I was always intrigued by the idea of translational medicine-bench to bedside and community medicine. The process of applying knowledge from basic biology and clinical trials to techniques and tools that address critical medical needs has always interested me. The KRISP labs are situated in the CAPRISA building right next to our university. CAPRISA (the Centre for the AIDS Programme of Research in South Africa) was home to some of the most advanced cutting-edge technology for biochemical research on our continent. Doctors from some of the world's top universities worked there and formed an incredible think tank. If I was going to get lab work done, my best bet was to join CAPRISA and KRISP.

One day, I Googled KRISP labs and sent them an e-mail (another example of the importance of being curious and trying new things). One of the heads of the labs-Veron Ramsuran-started mentoring me in the ways of genetics research. The rest is history. Using many of the skills that I learned in the genetics labs, I have been able to better understand how clinical research works and how I can use those skills to help our communities. For example, through KRISP, I completed a bioinformatics course which deepened my understanding of making phylogenetic trees (a sort of family tree that can help track evolutionary relationships between things). That skill helped me design a tree for COVID-19 when our world was struck by a pandemic in 2020 (more on that later). I used it to reassure people that the COVID-19 virus was not significantly mutating when the outbreak started. Finding ways to research relevant problems is a skill that I think every student should cultivate.

Innovation in medical research is exceptionally important and I advise all members of the healthcare multidisciplinary team to stay ahead of the game and innovate where possible. The lessons about curiosity and asking for help that I reinforced during my pediatrics block helped me in this regard. Seeing the implementation of research in such a way that it directly impacts people in a community is incredibly fulfilling. The primary health care block reinforced my appreciation for this feeling of fulfillment, by giving me many chances to get to know patients very intimately.

INTERNAL MEDICINE

Bringing everything together

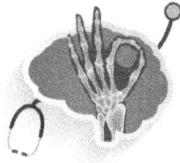

"The practice of medicine is an art, not a trade; a calling, not a business; a calling in which your heart will be exercised equally with your head."

— *WILLIAM OSLER*

Internal medicine is usually the first thing that people think about when they hear the word:" doctor." Imagine setting up drips, giving injections, working out diagnoses and looking at X-rays pensively. Grey's Anatomy eat your heart out. For the final clinical rotation of my 4th year of medical school; I returned to Prince Mshiyeni hospital. I have grown fond of that hospital. The staff are friendly and you get a great workout by walking from one ward to the next. I spent the final 12 weeks of 2019 there, in the internal medicine department. The hospital is semi-rural and is surrounded by informal settlements that spill over into the hospital premises. The drive to Prince Mshiyeni hospital from my home usually lasted about 40 minutes, with traffic. Those lengthy commutes along the N3 (national highway) allowed me enough time to reflect on how much I had transformed, during that year. Transformation and adaptability is an important part of the healing process.

I remember my first day of medical school very clearly. I was seated with about 250 of my first-year classmates, in L7 (the name of the lecture venue for first-year students), which was newly built. Everything in L7 was new and clean. You could see your reflection in the tiers of polished wooden desks. Most of us were fresh out of high school, with textbooks in one hand and coffee in the other. We were all so excited to start a new journey in our lives, make new friends, and save the world in our crisp new white lab coats.

Medical school changes us in many ways. 6 years is a long time to study for a degree. Many of us have transformed. Our bodies are in a constant state of change. Many of our cells undergo frequent turnover. After about 6 years; many of our cells are completely replaced. Our social, economic, cultural, and personal experiences also change us drastically. I can tell you that I am not the same person I was, on the first day of medical school. But, as I mentioned earlier, we must maintain the enthusiasm of our first-year selves, if we hope to be happy in our line of work. Many of my experiences in medical school have made me more resilient. The traumas we face thicken our skin. This resilience is critical if we wish to muster the strength that is needed to save others. When you spend so much time away from your family, when your heart is broken or when you are starving after a call that seems to stretch on forever; resilience, endurance, and willpower become essential.

Love for my patients, my work, my colleagues, and the important people in my life, help me maintain this resilience. When we work towards an ideal version of ourselves-the type of person we wanted to be when we started studying medicine-every challenge becomes a new stepping-stone to greater things. Our bodies adapt.

And that is what I love about internal medicine. Every single cell that constitutes us is continuously changing and adapting to our circumstances. Our muscles grow when we exercise. New connections form in our brains when we learn something new. The design of the human body and all its systems is a work of beauty. Every organ system works with an incredible harmony that is the product of millions of years of evolution. Studying these systems and the genius behind them feels like a stat IV dose of concentrated passion. Adaptability is important in hospitals like Prince Mshiyeni, where resources are often limited. One needs to find clever and efficient solutions to survive there. For example, the hallways of Prince Mshiyeni are notoriously long. I even heard that one of the interns there used a skateboard to help him travel between wards quicker. Doctors used blankets to bind fractured pelvises when actual pelvic binders where unavailable. The squishy IV bags were used to help support the heads of patients with suspected spinal injuries. Running to the internal medicine wards there, often took up a good few minutes of my morning. There were more than 6 different wards, each filled with rows of bed-bound patients. It was not uncommon to find the corpses of patients from the previous night, in body bags at the ward entrance. Our views of death change, the more we see it. We become almost inured to it. We become more accepting of it, even though we fight against it. That is just another way we adapt.

I found some fascinating and rare clinical signs on my patients, while there. Clinical signs are clues that we find during our clinical examination of patients. If you get excited by finding these clues, internal medicine may be the discipline for you… Sherlock Holmes. Tuberculosis and HIV were the most common pathologies in the ward. I encountered an obtunded patient with Janeway lesions-an exceptionally rare clinical sign in the form of small red bumps on the palms or soles of patients with a disease called infective endocarditis-infection of the inner layer of the heart. The sign became very rare when antibiotics became widely accessible. Most of our consultants had never seen the sign before, despite learning about it in medical school. One of our professors quipped that if we ever saw a patient with that sign, he would personally co-author an academic paper with us. The patient passed away before I could see him again. Within a few hours, the bed was filled with a new patient. That is just the way public hospitals have to operate, if they want to meet the patient caseload...

Most of our time was spent taking histories from the patients, examining them, and presenting them to our consultants, who were often strict, but they meant well. They were a wellspring of clinical knowledge. We also spent time attending dermatology tutorials (where we saw countless patients with acne) or visiting the hospital clinic and emergency room to assist the other doctors. A useful tip that we all learned was to befriend the nurses. They are usually the most experienced people in the wards when it comes to doing procedures like inserting IV lines or taking blood for laboratory analysis, which forms the bulk of our work during our internship years. Observing their skills and helping them are incredibly valuable learning opportunities for students.

Time in the internal medicine wards also gave us the chance to refine some of our more challenging procedural skills, such as lumbar punctures (where you insert a needle into a patient's spine to collect their spinal fluid), urethral catheterization (where you collect urine by passing a tube into a patient's urethra and thereafter pushing it into his/her bladder) and lymph node biopsies (taking out part of a patient's lymph node, to see if it may be affected by diseases). These procedures can be scary for both the student and the patient especially when you attempt them for the first time.

Many students love internal medicine because of how cerebral the subject is. I met a surgeon who joked that surgeons can do everything, but know nothing versus internists who know everything but can do nothing.

I love the thrill of discussing a patient's history, clinical examination findings, and investigation results, to come up with a diagnosis and then help manage the patient accordingly. I feel like a detective whenever I do it. Internal medicine makes you realize how vast medicine is. There is an amazing rush that one experiences, whenever one has a revelatory flash of diagnostic skill-when one puts all the pieces of the puzzle together and unveils the patient's diagnoses. Sometimes, the process is slower and should be savored, like enjoying a fine wine. Many doctors dream of being master diagnosticians. It is a vivifying and addictive feeling. Of course, one does not always have the luxury of time, when diagnosing patients, especially in the emergency room.

Working in the emergency room was...chaotic. We usually started our intake there at 4:00 pm on certain days and assisted the doctors until 10:00 pm. The entire hospital takes on a different atmosphere at night. On some nights, we were overwhelmed by waves of new patients. Sometimes, we saw no new patients at all. Because of limited resources, my colleagues and I often spent time scouring other medical rooms for equipment, including the one available ECG machine (a machine that can help us diagnose a lot of heart diseases). The doctors prayed that it kept working. It was battered after being pushed around the hospital so many times. A few of the electrodes were damaged.

Pandemonium reigned on some nights. You never know what you will see in the emergency room. I helped resuscitate a patient, which was an adrenaline rush. Our CPR instructors were fond of saying: "Every second lost is oxygen lost. I helped ventilate the patient while the senior doctors did the chest compressions. There was a time when a psychiatric patient threatened to stab all of us in the room before we surrounded him and the security guards pinned him down. We had to administer activated charcoal to a girl who ingested a poison. She was covered in the dark powder. These were just a few of many thrilling cases that we saw. The emergency room was an electrifying place, filled with patients as well as the doctors and nurses who helped them rage against the dying of the light.

I also witnessed my first patient death there...

She was an elderly woman who the doctors bravely tried to resuscitate, in her final few minutes of life. Her stillness felt unreal. It was my first time seeing an adult person completely motionless. The absence of a person's rhythmic rise and fall of the chest is eerily noticeable. Seeing a death for the first time feels like a rite of passage for any medical student. It is not as dramatic as Hollywood makes it seem. For some, it is a slow stepwise deterioration of human physiology, like falling through a series of the trapdoors-one system fails, then another. Multiple systems may fail. For some, it is a peaceful process. For others, they become restless and delirious. It is a complex process that made me reflect on my mortality and the importance of appreciating life, while we have it.

I saw, firsthand, the extremes of human physiology. I saw humans who were pushed to their limits-dying patients and the fervent, vigilant healthcare workers who helped bring them back from the brink. It was an incredible display of how every cell that makes us human, every organ system that orchestrates our survival, helps us resist anything, which tries to take precious life away from us.

I wrote this next article in light of my experiences in the internal medicine wards and the emergency room at Prince Mshiyeni.

RESISTANCE

My blood was slowly dripping, from my fists, onto the floor of our Kung Fu dojo at the Chinese Martial Arts and Health Centre in Durban. During iron body training, this is not an uncommon sight. It is a subset discipline within Shaolin Kung Fu that demands that martial arts students subject themselves to frequent and intense exercises (like agonizing knuckle pushups) to harden the body-if it is not difficult, if it is not challenging, there can be no transformation. This principle applies to almost every living organism, from bacteria...to medical students.

My colleagues and I completed our fourth year of medical school in October 2019. All of us braved the gauntlet of long work hours, relentless studying, irritable healthcare staff, and numerous other stressors in our personal lives. Many of us are not the same people we were at the beginning of that year.

Completing another year of medical school, like so many other goals in our work-a-day-world reminds me of the story of Sisyphus-a Greek king whose eternal punishment was to push a large boulder up a steep hill, only to repeat the arduous task, upon reaching the peak. Examining patients from 8:00 am to 4:00 pm (and even longer during hospital intakes) in the same healthcare setting ad infinitum can make many students and doctors empathize with Sisyphus who fought an unending uphill battle.

But is Sisyphus not stronger every time he lays his weary arms upon his burden?

Antimicrobial resistance is a phrase that has become terrifyingly common in healthcare settings. Many microorganisms, such as bacteria, are surviving our strongest pharmacological weapons. Extremely drug-resistant tuberculosis and multiple drug-resistant tuberculosis are persistent problems in South Africa that can be extraordinarily difficult to treat. The outcome can be fatal for many patients.

As medical students, we will soon be at the forefront of this antimicrobial resistance epidemic. It is crucial to identify, adjust and implement new strategies before we find ourselves unable to treat simple infections or unable to carry out simple procedures like abscess drainage or suturing of superficial wounds without running the risk of deadly consequences. Our greatest weapons against diseases might not work in the future. Many mosquitoes which spread malaria around the world have already become resistant to a drug called chloroquine, for example. Malaria claims millions of lives every year.

Some bacteria have an intrinsic, genetically determined resistance to antibiotics (intrinsic resistance-which is always expressed in the bacterial species and does not need to be induced by antibiotics). Or they may have induced resistance: The genes for resistance are present, but become expressed to resistance levels after exposure to antibiotics)-the antibiotics induce resistance. Other bacteria (known as persisters) naturally resist antibiotics but do not transfer this resistance to their offspring. It is interesting to think that some medical students are naturally resistant to the pressures of medical school and excel despite the onslaught of new stressors, in their personal and professional lives. There are stories of people who are naturally gifted and instinctually overcome all challenges in medical school, which remind me of the few bacteria that are created with an innate resistance to antibiotics. However, I feel that it is more interesting to talk about the bacteria and medical students that acquire resistance. Bacteria are a part of us and can be found all over us, even in our guts and on our skin. We share intimate relationships with them.

Bacteria develop resistance, by mutating to adapt to their environment or they acquire it from each other...much like us humans.

Bacteria exchange genetic material with each other through various means (called horizontal gene transfer). One way is through transformation-they absorb the DNA of their fallen comrades and learn from the failures and successes of others, much like medical students who ask their mentors for advice about the trials and tribulations of medical school.

Conjugation is another method, in which bacteria get together and say: "Hey I know ways to help you reproduce better. So, let's have sex to exchange information." I imagine that this way of transferring information is not as common as the others, among medical students...

Through many of these mechanisms; bacteria and medical students become stronger. Bacteria learn to decrease drug uptakes, modify drug targets, inactivate drugs, or push drugs out of them. Medical students learn to deal with common stressors (such as high workload, performance pressure, conflict with faculty, time constraints, peer relations and their social environment, heartbreak, career planning and concerns about the future, financial concerns...the list goes on) as time passes. It is easy to feel as if one is drowning. Many of us have different coping strategies (exercise, reading, extracurricular activities, socializing, hobbies). The Red Queen Hypothesis applies to both us as students and bacteria-we must constantly adapt and evolve to survive, while pitted against ever-evolving opposing organisms in a constantly changing environment. We are running on a treadmill to stay in the same place...but we become stronger purely because we are running, no matter how exhausting it may seem.

The fact that there are happy doctors out there, even in resource-limited settings, is living proof that there are people who are resistant to these stressors (as well as others). It is also possible that they developed resistance over time.

We could reflect upon our first-year selves and see someone completely different. We could reflect upon whom we were at the start of this year and see someone completely different as well.

Some may collapse under these new stressors and some may very well excel in other environments. Some rise to the challenges of our crucible. They endure great pain and are tempered in its fires. They see these emotional micro-fractures as iron body training for the soul-a Sisyphus who is stronger every time he pushes the boulder- a student or doctor who is stronger with each passing year.

Witnessing a death for the first time, in the emergency room also compelled me to contemplate how we view death in society. Again, I was reminded of the phrase "Mono no aware"-which means, "the pathos of things" -a melancholic appreciation of the transience of existence (the bittersweetness of things).

Patient deaths remind of my adventures in China, India, and Nepal, during December 2016. During my journey, I ventured to rural China, where my family and I embarked on a cruise along the Yangtze River. The beauty of that place still brings tears to my eyes. One of our destinations was Fengdu, which is believed by the people who live there, to be the manifestation of the Chinese underworld-the city of death. My perspective of the transience of life and the paths that lead all living things to their end was changed in that sacred place.

When we entered the city, we were required to pass several tests, which challenge the soul. My time there also allowed me a valuable chance to reflect on my understanding of disease, my research with CAPRISA and the KRISP genetics labs as well as how our work impacts life and death.

My travels through rural China as well as rural India, Russia, South America, Europe, Japan, and South Africa also exposed me to many traditional medicines and health practices which have inspired me and have broadened my view of medicine. I learned to love a South American herbal tea called Yerba mate, which apparently contains many antioxidants. Many years ago, I was asked by a few Chinese tourists if I was studying Western or Eastern medicine. I had never been asked that question before. In South Africa, we usually just say that we study medicine (as if Western medicine encompasses everything about medicine). We often forget that many of our remedies are derived from plants and traditional medicines. My adventures abroad have reminded me of the importance of learning from other cultures, maintaining our connection to nature, and collaborating with traditional medicine healers/practitioners who offer wisdom, which we may not learn in Western medical schools. In the White Emperor City along the Yangtze River, I saw community members gather in a circle every evening at a designated spot, to dance to traditional music, learn traditional martial arts like tai chi, exchange home remedies, socialize and exercise for good health. The community members attended those gatherings religiously. Traditions that promoted health were eagerly embraced by them. Even now, I can still remember their dance moves. It was a moving experience.

My travels have taught me that medicine is universal. It is not an isolated discipline. It has a long legacy that has been developed through shared human knowledge. Our traditions are an example of this. Many of my family members still prefer to use traditional Ayurvedic medicines. My Kung Fu instructor showed me how to use a homemade Taiwanese ointment for wounds and joint pain caused by our martial arts training. My father received an honorary professorship for supporting traditional healers in our province. Many of our traditional healers still believe in magic and umuthi (traditional medicine) for attracting good luck or warding off evil spirits. While learning about palliative care, we were taught about alternative non-pharmacological measures of pain control like aromatherapy, acupuncture, or music therapy. I had the privilege of meeting some Israeli women who had finished their military service. One of the women was trained in music therapy. My brother and I joined one of her therapy sessions with a few of our friends from Japan. We all played various instruments, while one of the ladies sang a traditional Israeli song. She encouraged us to make our own rhythms and melodies to add to her songs. Playing the guitar in tandem with her singing felt liberating and calming. As a pianist, I have noticed that medicine is filled with different rhythms and melodies. The heartbeat is a rhythm. Our brainwaves follow patterns. Even our sleep cycles work according to so called: "circadian rhythms". Disruptions in our rhythms can impair our wellbeing. Music can help us correct these imbalances.

I owe much to the people who I have met throughout my travels and I am grateful to my dad for allowing me to explore the world. Learning more about people has greatly expanded my views of medicine and different modalities of treatment.

THE KINGDOM OF SOULS

The air was lavishly perfumed with rain when our boat docked at the misty harbor of the city of ghosts in December 2016. A wave of unease swept over my fellow passengers, as we gazed at the proud rock sculpture before us-the head of The Ghost King, whose proud visage was carved into a nearby mountain.

Fengdu, a mysterious 2000-year-old city was our port of call for the day-a rest stop on our journey along the mighty Yangtze River. After breakfast, we ventured to an ancient hilltop temple complex, where I was faced with my first test of the soul. The temples were shrouded in mist. It was a scene straight out of an epic Kung Fu movie. Some Chinese people believe that Fengdu is the final destination of all human spirits, that have left our mortal world. The souls must pass three tests, to vanish into the afterlife. I stood at the site of the first test: Tianzi Palace, where one must choose to cross only one of two bridges: The bridge of health or the bridge of wealth.

As a medical student in South Africa, a developing country with steadily rising unemployment as well as TB, and HIV prevalence rates; I have seen that the paths to either of these two bridges are undulating and often obstructed. Inequality and poverty are monolithic barriers to improvements in global health. Tuberculosis, the White plague, the pathological extreme of Victorian romanticism, is fueled by these two products of Pandora's box. South Africa, my home, maintains one of the highest TB and HIV burdens in the world.

In 2016, while also sightseeing in the vibrant streets of Goa, India; I was shaken by a sudden, piercing cry-a a woman's tortured bloodcurdling shriek-that erupted from a nearby dilapidated building. Several walls had collapsed and the floors were covered in dust, glass and rubble. I could hear many people coughing inside the building. I later learned that it was a TB hospital. The woman's scream still haunts me.

That first test also reminded me of a quote by Mahatma Gandhi: "It is health that is real wealth and not pieces of gold and silver." In our profession, there is a stereotype that all doctors are paid well. This largely depends on which specialty one chooses. In many cases, doctors in specialties that require procedural sills (e.g., surgery), tend to earn better than those who do not perform procedural skills. This is not a hard and fast rule. Some general practitioners in South Africa earn very well and sometimes earn more than specialists. Yes, it is important to earn well and doctors tend to have great financial security, which is a good reason for pursuing a job in medicine. But I do not think that it should be the only reason. I have known people who claimed that they only studied medicine because of potential financial gain and the status that accompanies the title of being a doctor (being a doctor can also help your romantic prospects). Many of them were often highly unsatisfied with their work. When you work a 48-hour shift in a busy hospital, you have to love what you do, if you want to stay sane in this field. There are some important questions to ask yourself when studying medicine. Can you enjoy doing it for the rest of your life? Can you be financially secure and attain your financial goals? Will you still have enough time for the people and things that matter to you? Wealth is only one of many factors that must be considered, before one can walk across the bridge of health. It cannot be the only factor, if you choose to stay healthy.

The second test of the soul lay ahead of us...the test of strength. A heavy stone weight lay within a smooth pit, carved into the earth. To pass this test; we were required to remove the weight from the pit. Many of us nearly broke our backs trying to heave the stone out of its pit. An elderly farmer silently observed us. Eventually, he shuffled over to the steadfast rock...and started rolling it. He used the momentum of the weight to gently push it out of its pit. It was a test of the brain, not brawn.

TB persists in many developing countries for many reasons (e.g., overcrowding and the emergence of antibiotic-resistant mycobacterial strains). It has become apparent that bombarding TB with a pharmacopeia of drugs is the equivalent to using brute force to pass the test of strength. Smart, simple, and innovative solutions are the real source of our diagnostic and therapeutic powers.

It was this same reasoning that led me to the KRISP organization (KwaZulu Natal Research and Innovation Sequencing Platform), a titan in the world of TB and HIV genetics research. Application forms for a polymerase chain reaction (PCR) course were posted on their website. The opportunity to elucidate TB through this revolutionary biochemical technique was irresistible. Much like the fire of Prometheus that was bestowed upon us; PCR has given us previously unobtainable power-the ability to exponentially amplify DNA-the entity that binds me to the woman in Goa and every other living organism.

During the course, we learned about the seemingly limitless uses of this technique: genetic cloning and sequencing, PCR-based DNA fingerprinting for forensic analysis, and even the precise identification of the organisms that cause TB. Amplifying DNA in the cutting-edge gene Xpert and thermocycler devices, like those at KRISP, has allowed for faster, cheaper, and more accurate point-of-care diagnoses for many diseases, even in primary healthcare centers, where poorer patients can receive cutting-edge treatment-thus supporting the principles of an inclusive society. Perhaps, someday, we can attain instant, affordable, and completely precise diagnoses for all diseases, with this technique. It feels empowering to use the skills that we read about in textbooks.

The final test challenges the soul to stand atop a smooth rock (a representation of balance in life and death). I was reminded of the importance of staying balanced in life when studying medicine. I caught another glimpse of the, "mortal world," before I prepared to, "accept my fate and pass into the afterlife" according to our tour guide. Seeing life from the perspective of the dead reminds us that life is precious and often unbalanced. Innovations in science and medicine, like PCR, profoundly influence the eternal conflict between illness and health, to make our journey through life...and into the afterlife, much easier.

SURGERY

A sharp blade demands a sharp mind

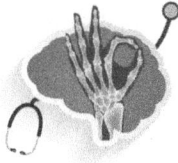

"Surgeons must be very careful

When they take the knife!

Underneath their fine incisions

Stirs the Culprit—Life!"

— *EMILY DICKINSON*

The year was 2020, the start of my 5th and penultimate year of medical school. I had just returned from Japan (where my brother and I trained with ninja and samurai) and South Korea-two of the first few countries that were invaded by a virus that brought the entire world to a grinding halt. During my time in the east and my time reading the teachings of Miyamoto Musashi and Sun Tzu, I developed a much greater respect for the sword and other blades. The samurai master who taught us was a short and intensely focused Japanese man. He inherited a 700-year-old blade that was passed down through many generations of his family. He demonstrated his skills for us and then taught my brother and me how to wield the blade. It could cut bamboo and bone like butter…

Much like surgeons, the samurai could decide life and death with their blades. Our samurai master taught us to perform a prayer, before ever wielding a blade, out of respect for the power that it gives us. He reminded us that the samurai's purpose is to serve and to protect. The code that they follow-Bushido is a set of guidelines that recommend how samurai should behave. It shares some common elements with the professional guidelines that we follow as doctors (especially regarding honesty, justice, character, and self-control). The surgeon, much like the samurai, uses the blade to serve society, by defending society from diseases. It was fascinating to see how the philosophies from one ancient Eastern art translated to another ancient Western art. My samurai master and my surgery lecturers told me the same thing: "A true master knows when not to cut."

5th-year UKZN medical students are trained in Pietermaritzburg hospitals, as part of a decentralized clinical training program that was established by our university and our provincial department of health.

I wrote about my experiences in the surgery department in the following article that I published with the Harvard Medical School Review journal.

SURGERY IN THE TIME OF COVID-19

Our first clinical rotation for 2020 was surgery, at Grey's Hospital-the main tertiary hospital in Pietermaritzburg and the surrounding areas. Pietermaritzburg is a peaceful and verdant town in the province of KwaZulu Natal, about a 1-hour drive away from Durban-my home city. The air is cool and fresh there and the hills seem to roll on forever.

During our 7-week surgical block, we rotated through general surgery, ophthalmology, ENT, urology, and orthopedics. The urologists love good humor. We needed to attend at least four intakes during that time (during which we would need to work in the emergency room and the surgical wards from 8:00 am-10:00 pm -which was an incredible memory for me).

We were five weeks into our surgical block when we received news that COVID-19 had reached South Africa. Our university quickly established a war room, where a select group of doctors and scientists could help prepare us for this new public health threat. Many of the scientists worked with CAPRISA. Grey's Hospital turned part of its maternity ward into an isolation unit for patients who were infected. We were trained in the management of COVID-19 patients within a few days. However, everyone was still nervous. Our country has an incredibly high burden of HIV and TB, and many of our public health hospitals were reeling under the pressure of high patient caseloads at baseline. It was the perfect storm for a health crisis that would shake our nation to its core.

Many of the medical students left our first COVID-19 training session with a sense of growing anticipation. When the training finished, night had fallen and the temperature plummeted. I took a deep breath and gazed over the valleys of pine trees that surrounded the hospital. The fog was approaching. It was just a matter of time before it engulfed us.

I have had the privilege of working in every public hospital in my home city. Many of these facilities lack sufficient personal protective equipment for doctors and the medical equipment (e.g., ventilators) and beds that were needed to meet the daily needs of patients. The slowly rising number of COVID-19 cases galvanized our department of health into action. Hospitals throughout the country converted wards into isolation units. Field hospitals were established in our World Cup stadiums and mobile testing clinics were deployed to relieve overwhelmed public health facilities. Our country was preparing for a national State of Disaster…and we were in the dark.

Within two weeks, the South African government made a historical decision to institute a nationwide lockdown. We were seeing a new chapter in history unfolding before our very eyes. On the 15th of March, our university withdrew all the medical students from their clinical rotations. We had so many questions. We did not know if we would finish our year on time. Many students could not access online lectures or submit assignments, owing to a lack of Wi-Fi, in rural areas. We were confused and unsettled. I was at my aunt's house in Durban when we heard the president's address. My aunt's immediate response was to hoard hand sanitizer and stockpile food and water. She was distraught. I tried to calm her down, but to be honest…I was struggling to suppress my anxiety.

On the first morning of lockdown, I awoke to the sound of silent streets--a first for Durban. If you listened closely, you could even hear birdsong--a welcome replacement for the usual cacophony of morning traffic.

Eventually, I worked out a daily quarantine routine. I tried to wake up at 8:30 am consistently. Most of my time involved reading my medical textbooks, completing my research, playing the piano, exercising, and chatting with my family. There is a beautiful bird, Hadeda ibis, which is native to Sub-Saharan Africa and commonly seen around Durban. They started nesting along the promenade, where I enjoy my evening jogs. I even started a medical-themed comedy web show, which served as my platform for educating the general public about COVID-19 and inspiring solidarity during those uncertain times.

Our university created a series of COVID-19-related epidemiology and bioinformatics webinars for medical doctors and scientists, which I enjoyed attending and then reformatting to communicate the information to a lay audience. I often used the, "Ask a Question" function on the social media platform Instagram to hear what my friends and family thought about those drastic changes in the world and our way of life. I received many questions like, "Is there a coronavirus cure?" or, "How long will it take to make a vaccine?" I did my best to answer them and allay their fears. Every era in history creates new fears and casts illness in its own image. Society, like the ultimate psychosomatic patient, matches its medical afflictions to its psychological crises. When a disease touches such a visceral chord, it is often because the chord is already resonating.

There are, however, many questions, which I could not answer, like, "Will the world ever be the same again?" or, "How do I overcome my fear of death by coronavirus?" Inspiring hope in others and fighting fear with education demands an act of exquisite measuring and remeasuring, filling and unfilling a psychological respirator with oxygen. I feel that it is an operation just as delicate and complex as the performance of surgery.

Everyone, except for essential workers, was required to remain at home for several weeks. Many countries around the world were starting to implement lockdowns as well. A new terrifying chapter of history was unfolding before our eyes. The global economy was bracing itself for one of the worst recessions in history. Business Insider dubbed it the "Great Lockdown" global recession-the worst recession since the Great Depression. The world was preparing for a war with a virus. Viruses are masters of the Art of War. My ninjitsu training in Japan, as well as my practice of medicine and bioinformatics, deepened my respect for viruses. While in quarantine, I compared the COVID-19 Coronavirus to the ninja under whom I also trained.

THE VIRAL ART OF WAR

Before the 2020 Coronavirus pandemic brought the world to a standstill; my twin brother and I ventured to Japan to learn the arts of the ninja. It was during December, 2019-our third visit to Japan and our first visit to South Korea-when the Coronavirus was still emerging in a wet animal market in Wuhan city, China. Those three countries were the first to fall victim to the pandemic. We witnessed the calm just before the storm-a world oblivious to a war that would be waged by a virus.

Our adventures lead us to Kyoto, the ancient capital of Japan, where we met a master of ninjitsu, in an inconspicuous dojo on 528 Hakurakutencho Street. When we entered, there was no one to be seen. We admired the rows of swords, sickles, brass knuckles, and blowguns that lined the walls.

"I see you are here for your training session."

We spun around, surprised by the deep voice that interrupted our awe. Our ninja master had materialized from the shadows and caught us unawares. He looked like a Japanese version of Johnny Depp, with long jet-black hair. He appeared relaxed and smiled often, but his sharp features and piercing gaze were unnerving. I could not help but feel both fascinated and cautious.

My interest in ninjitsu stems from my practice of martial arts, such as Kung Fu, at the Durban Chinese Martial Arts and Health Centre in KwaZulu Natal.

Our master taught us that ninja were specialized assassins, saboteurs, and secret agents of medieval Japanese warfare, who were trained in the arts of espionage, deception, and strategy. The earliest reports of their existence were made in the 15th Century (during the Japanese Warring States Period) when ninjas were required for reconnaissance and disruption of enemy forces.

My brother and I were trained in the use of some of the more commonly used traditional shinobi weapons-such as the kusarigama (crescent-shaped sickle), hokode (sharpened claws for offense and scaling walls), blowgun, and makibishi (sharp metal traps for impeding a pursuing enemy).

Espionage training followed. We were taught evasive maneuvers, silent walking techniques, the disarming of enemies, and the use of traps.

What amazed me the most about the ninja was their versatility. Survival and espionage are of utmost importance to the shinobi. They were taught athletics, martial arts, topography, the use of fire and medicine, along with a myriad of other skills to help them adapt to almost any situation.

According to Sun Tzu's legendary military text, "The Art of War: "All warfare is based on deception." The ninjas excelled at this and were often feared as supernatural beings. Luring the enemy into a false sense of security, striking at critical moments, displaying adaptability, and disrupting the enemy are hallmarks of strategic warfare. I have seen these core tactics being employed in Kung Fu and Ninjitsu.

As a medical student…I see it in viruses as well.

When the South African government first implemented a nationwide quarantine to control the spread of Coronavirus; I could not help but spare some time to appreciate the elegance of the Coronavirus design. I used some of the bioinformatics skills that I acquired from the genetics experts at KRISP to investigate this new threat further.

The COVID-19 Coronavirus is a spherical or pleomorphic enveloped particle, with membrane proteins, that contains single-stranded (positive sense) RNA, with a nucleoprotein within a capsid comprised of matrix protein. It resembles a ball with spikes. Its design is morbidly beautiful. The fact that this microorganism brought the world to its knees is incredible. Within two months, it spread to the rest of the planet, while sabotaging our immune systems. It silently ambushes its victims. It sews panic into society and galvanizes the spread of misinformation (fake news). Viruses are masters of the art of war. Viruses use many tools and weapons (virulence factors) much like ninjas, to infect us.

"Corona" means, "crown", in Latin. Coronavirus resembles a crown when viewed through an electron microscope. We can see it and study it. Unveiling the virus reveals its weaknesses. We take the ninja out of the shadows.

Sun Tzu also states," "Know the enemy and know yourself; in a hundred battles, you will never be in peril." Every day during our national lockdown, we discovered new strategies to beat this virus. The KRISP labs created new genome detection tools. New antiviral drugs were tested. Vaccine development progressed faster than ever. Educating the public about the virus- teaching others to know the enemy and understand the enemy's weaknesses- (e.g., frequent hand washing, improved hygiene practices, and social distancing) were critical strategies for beating the virus. I did this by hosting a medical-themed web show and by blogging about my experiences and research findings in the hope that I could educate others and inspire solidarity during those uncertain times. Medical communication is my weapon of choice.

I was just about to finish my 5th-year surgical rotation at Grey's Hospital, in the peaceful town of Pietermaritzburg, before the quarantine started. Our routines changed, yet we adapted to those new situations. Every day, my fellow medical students and I revised our coursework, exercised, volunteered, and helped collect data for our healthcare workers and researchers who fought tirelessly at the front line. We could not allow others to be caught unawares. We united to clear the shadows.

When the COVID-19 pandemic started, the world experienced a paradigm shift. Being isolated from my patients and my friends awakened something within me. I thought to myself: "I cannot just sit around and wait for the world to restart." There was much talk about a "new normal" in the world. People were starting to realize that our old way of doing things (e.g., shaking hands and lenient hygiene rules) needed to change if we wanted to prevent a pandemic like that from rearing its head in the future.

Many countries around the world, including South Africa, instituted quarantine measures to slow down the spread of COVID-19. There were 5 stages to the lockdown. Only certain people who provided, "essential services (e.g., qualified healthcare workers and emergency service workers) were permitted to leave their homes. Non-essential workers and other people could only leave their homes to acquire necessities (e.g., groceries or healthcare services).

I could not help but wonder what COVID-19 patients were enduring in hospitals. Most of the information that we were hearing about them came from sensational news reports on TV, that instilled panic and anxiety in many.

But I saw this as an opportunity.

Most news shows were portraying the serious and often terrifying view of COVID-19. I used my Instagram account to ask my friends what they thought about the new pandemic. Many of them felt that their fear of the virus stemmed from a lack of understanding about the virus and how one can protect oneself against it.

I have always been a fan of acting and great movies. Getting into character and imitating the behaviors of others requires keen observational skills and great empathy. I even studied drama as one of my subjects in high school. While I was in Japan a few months before the pandemic started, I purchased a tripod stand from an amazing (and incredibly eccentric) convenience store called Don Quixote. The electronics section was right next to the sex toy section. I thought that I could combine my medical knowledge of the virus (which I obtained mainly by attending online COVID-19 training courses and conferences with the KRISP labs) with my acting skills, to raise awareness about COVID-19 entertainingly. So, one day, I suited up, wrote a script, and started my own YouTube show, which I dubbed, "The Quarantine Show." In the show, I turned COVID-19 into a character, who I interviewed, in a Jimmy Fallon-esque style. When I started sharing my videos on social media, it became fairly popular amongst my friends and family. Eventually, a local TV station contacted me, interviewed me, and asked me to be a voice-over artist and TV presenter on their show, "African Essence." I then started using this platform to help raise awareness about important social issues in South Africa (e.g., domestic abuse, mental health disorders, and organ trafficking). It was a great example of how one can turn any situation into something positive by combining different skills. You can create something novel and unexpected, that could help many people. Through African Essence, I met some amazing young people with a flair for TV presenting. Together, we covered episodes about salient social topics like prostitution in Durban, domestic abuse/violence, human interest stories during the lockdown, crime as well as many other important discussion points that deepened my understanding of the social determinants of health in my city. We had sobering discussions with drug abusers, police, prostitutes, victims of crime, local celebrities, doctors and many other people from all walks of life. My work with African Essence also allowed me to act in local films, which was a great deal of fun. Entertainment is a powerful tool for getting people to become interested in something.

I wanted so desperately to raise awareness of the virus. I know what it feels like to be stuck in a hospital ward for days on end, with a respiratory condition. I could only imagine what COVID-19 patients must have experienced. I recalled one of my childhood illnesses to try to empathize with them better.

THAT OTHER PLACE

"Illness is the night-side of life, a more onerous citizenship. Everyone who is born holds dual citizenship, in the kingdom of the well and the kingdom of the sick. Although we all prefer to use only the good passport, sooner or later each of us is obliged, at least for a spell, to identify ourselves as citizens of that other place."

— *SUSAN SONTAG*

During 2011, I fell ill with a case of pneumonia, during a family vacation, on a cruise ship, off the coast of Italy. I was rushed to the nearest pediatric hospital at the next port of call in Naples. My memories of that holiday are fragmented, but my recollection of my illness is crystal clear. Throughout my medical training, I have met countless people-each with their unique approaches to dealing with adversity and the recovery process. My 5 years of medical training, coupled with thousands of hours of learning about diseases from books and ward rounds have strengthened the empathy that I feel for my patients. But I learned long ago, in my hospital bed in Naples, that the best way to learn about a disease and the people who are afflicted by it, is to experience it first-hand. Disease is the best teacher about disease.

Naples has beautiful warm weather, sparkling seas and a rich history. I was admitted to an incredibly comfortable pediatric ward on the second floor of the hospital. The hallways were colorful and decorated with pictures of Disney characters. It was a warm and inviting atmosphere for any child-including me, the only non-Italian patient in the entire hospital, at the time.

I learned that it was rare for foreigners to be admitted to that small Italian hospital. Some of the more curious nurses occasionally stopped at my room to catch a glimpse of me and wave. Smiling and hand gestures were my only means of communication, even with the young girl with whom I shared my room.

When she was first admitted to the ward, we bonded immediately-over our respiratory illnesses. She was incredibly sweet and her face was constantly illuminated by a broad smile. We spoke to each other using broken English. Sarah (not her real name) lived in Naples with her parents, who visited her daily. They were jovial people who were all-too-willing to share their home-cooked meals with us (including irresistible asparagus and Parma ham sandwiches which remain etched into my memory). We all grew closer during the week of my hospital stay.

When I wasn't playing with Sarah, I tried to find other ways to keep myself occupied. I quickly finished reading the only book that I had with me at the time, "Harry Potter and the Goblet of Fire." The hours pass slowly when one is a patient. Every day, you wake up to see the same 4 white walls and follow a strict treatment regimen. If there was anything, besides talking to Sarah, that raised my spirits, it was the amazing hospital food. To this day, I have never tasted better Italian food. The carbonara pasta was to die for. The hospital was catered for by a popular local restaurant. It is easy to lose track of time when the only thing you wait for is a daily hospital visit from your family or a delicious meal. A week in that hospital felt like a month, even though I had a very pleasant experience there. I often think about my patients who receive neither family visits nor tasty meals. What else do they look forward to in the day, while they soldier through their predictable treatment plans? I imagine that their hospital stays as well as their illnesses feel like they last much longer than they do. When patients ask me, "Will I be discharged today?" I understand their frustration.

At the time, I did not understand what pneumonia was. I had an inkling that it was some disease, caused by bacteria that infected the lungs. I wanted to know why the doctors often asked me to expectorate and describe the color of my sputum. What difference did it make? I worked out that rust-colored sputum was bad and that was something I should watch out for. Taking my antibiotics at a set time every day was a ritual that I transformed into a sort of game. I tried to memorize the names of the antibiotics and all the chemical names on the bottle, even though I didn't understand what they meant: Amoxicillin, azithromycin, ceftriaxone…

Ceftriaxone, brand name: Rocephin, is the one antibiotic that is highlighted most starkly in my memory. One of its routes of administration is through an intramuscular injection. The pain was excruciating. It usually left me in tears. I often pleaded with my dad to spare me the agony of that medication. The day I knew I would never forget Ceftriaxone, was when it was given to Sarah. Her screams were bloodcurdling…her pain was my pain.

There are many models of the patient-physician relationship, such as the patient-centered approach which views health care as, "closely congruent with and responsive to patients' wants, needs, and preferences or the paternalistic model, in which the physician is expected to best meet the health needs of assenting patients. However, there is justification for the equal consideration of equal interests in the physician-patient caring relationship: Moral rightness and mutual benefit. Biomedical ethics principles, moral reasoning, and public reasoning support the idea that patients and physicians have equal dignity and moral value because they are both moral agents. Physicians and patients are morally entitled-and according to their capacity-obliged to care and be cared about. Simply put, we must care about our doctors and our patients. You can't have one and not the other. Studies about reciprocation in caring suggest that it is likely to benefit both patients and physicians. Showing that you care is not just something that is nice to have. It makes everyone's lives better.

Some qualitative studies about medical students' and doctors' personal illness experiences suggest that medical students who choose to reflect on personal illness experiences have better empathy and respect for patients. Other qualitative studies suggest that doctors' self-reported," powerful experiences" followed by reflection and introspection, may lead to 'improved connectedness with others", or "increased productivity, energy or creativity." This, "improved connectedness with others" improves physician empathy for patients, which can improve patient care outcomes. Writing about our experiences and sharing them with others helps us connect with other people, which can improve how well we interact with our patients and other healthcare providers.

The social baseline theory (SBT) proposes that organisms are adapted to social ecology. Consequently, the social proximity to other individuals (characterized by familiarity, joint attention, shared goals, and interdependence) should be considered as the default or baseline assumption of the human brain.

Simply put, we are social beings.

Empirical studies on this theory have found that neural pathways and hormonal stress responses associated with self-regulation of emotion are less active when social support is provided or even anticipated. Several studies have shown that empathy and a supportive presence (even a photograph of a loved one) can decrease the feeling of pain. The Free Energy Principle proposed by Friston K. is an interesting explanation for why contextual and social factors, such as a clinician's empathy, may affect physical and mental health outcomes. I can attest to this. Having my dad around to comfort me, made injections feel somehow less painful. The tying of the tourniquet and the anticipation of the injection became part of my routine that I feared less and less over time.

I remember the feeling of the fresh sea air against my face when I left that hospital in Naples. It was a cathartic change from the stagnant hospital air. I still treasure many of my thoughts from that place-waking up to an Italian-style breakfast with fresh milk, the friendly nursing staff, and my dear friend Sarah. My time there fundamentally changed my view of disease and my understanding of the patient experience. Time seemed to pass so slowly there. I had more than enough time to reflect on my illness and the recovery process. My convalescence in Naples brought me closer to my patients.

Just as I prepared to leave my ward, Sarah rushed towards me and hugged me. There were tears in both of our eyes. We had barely spoken more than a few full sentences to each other, but our friendship had grown because of our illnesses. We knew what the other had endured. We were both citizens of that, "other place" and, despite all the coughing, crying, injections, and antibiotics, we returned home, with a bond that will last a lifetime.

During the COVID-19 pandemic, I asked myself the question: "why do we fear disease?" My work in the wards and the lab has deepened my appreciation for the great complexity of humans and the phenomena that interfere with our homeostasis. The Red Queen Hypothesis suggests that humans must evolve to adapt because we are competing with other evolving organisms, like viruses. This desire to propagate compelled me to consider the similarities between humans and viruses and imagine what would happen if the COVID-19 virus could speak and think like a human.

I do not believe that viruses or any other force of nature should be feared or labeled as intrinsically good or evil. Viruses are what they are. In the following article, "Coronation" that I wrote for an international medical essay competition, I chose to depict COVID-19 as a vulnerable and misunderstood monarch, that needs humans as much as a king needs his subjects (Corona means crown in Latin). By understanding the science behind diseases, we elucidate their weaknesses and help others realize that viruses should never be feared, but understood. Monarchs derive their power from their control over their subjects, much like how COVID-19 spreads because we choose to give it power over us. We can change this. I wanted to imagine what it would be like if the COVID-19 Coronavirus was a person.

As a medical writer, medical student, and TV presenter, I use my voice to educate others about the virus and help dispel the ignorance that helps it spread. As a future medical doctor, I dream of bridging the gap between the general public and medical science, by making medical pedagogy and communication accessible and entertaining for all. Fear can be replaced with knowledge. COVID-19 or any other disease should hold no dominion over us.

CORONATION

Every microorganism dreams of receiving the title: "pandemic"- the viral equivalent of a human coronation ceremony. I have been inspired by the stories of Spanish flu & swine flu-legendary viruses that traveled across the world and made millions of human friends.

When I first learned how to befriend the humans, they bestowed upon me the royal soubriquet: "COVID-19." It is a fitting title for a descendant of the distinguished order Nidovirales from the famous Coronaviridae family. I cannot resist flaunting my crown before the paparazzi and their electron microscopes.

To be honest, I'm still just a humble enveloped, positive-stranded RNA virus who loves crowded spaces, traveling by air, and multiplying ad infinitum. I owe much to my human friends who helped me achieve this glorious dream. They are incredibly accommodating hosts who offer me free, comfortable lodging in their warm airways. I would like to personally apologize for my progeny that have incited inflammatory responses in some humans. My children can be quite a handful.

Replicating inside humans affords me the luxury of hearing their thoughts about the viral monarchy. Apparently, I'm not very popular. Some are even contemplating a vaccine coup!

I don't understand. Humans are a confusing species. They need to reproduce to continue their lineage. The Red Queen hypothesis suggests that I must do the same.

Nonetheless, I will do my best to win over the humans. Black Death (a close friend of the royal family) kickstarted the Renaissance. It's not easy being king. I have much to do if I want to be remembered like my legendary pandemic predecessors...of course, that depends on the love and support that I receive from my human subjects.

Despite my efforts to understand the virus better and to protect myself from it, I was still infected by it. During December 2020, shortly after I finished my final exams, I fell ill with a fever and myalgia-soreness and aching in the muscles. It happened around

Christmas time. I feared the worst. When I received my test results and discovered that I was COVID positive, I felt angry… with myself. I felt careless. I had put my family at risk. After seeing so much suffering in the medical outpatient department, the last thing I wanted to do was subject my family and friends to the same burden.

For 2 weeks, I remained in isolation, at home, during the festive season. I saw it as an opportunity to familiarize myself with the virus on a more intimate level. I was reminded of the lockdown earlier that year. It is easy to lose track of time. The days flowed into each other. I spent much of my time writing, relaxing, and finding new ways to stay productive. I was glad that we had a balcony, from which I could watch over the city and reflect on everything that happened during my 5th year. Living in a new environment, away from home, reinforced my appreciation for my family as well as my ability to live independently. For many of us, COVID-19 had caused immense suffering. I knew people who had lost family members and businesses to the pandemic. Gender-based violence and mental health issues, like depression, were exacerbated by the lockdown. There was so much sorrow.

During my isolation, I reflected on the vulnerability of healthcare professionals. Some of our family friends who were frontline healthcare workers died because of the virus. Almost every day, we endure long working hours, high patient caseloads, and personal issues. There is always a risk of acquiring disease as well. An advantage of working in healthcare is that society seems to look up to us and respect our choices, most of the time. We also get sick. Sometimes, we make mistakes and we cannot save everyone. We adapt to our circumstances, but we are not perfect. I feel that accepting that we do make mistakes as humans and that we must continuously improve, despite our challenges, is an important step towards finding peace and psychological well-being in our profession.

My isolation reminded me of the importance of diversifying my skill set. David Epstein's research supports the idea of exploring a range of interests instead of overspecializing in a single field. He conveys this point in his thought-provoking book: "Range: Why Generalists Triumph in a Specialized World." I am a strong proponent of this idea. It reminds me of the memories of my dad pushing us to try many different activities. Even when studying medicine, I have never underestimated the value of exploring different interests and hobbies. Many of those hobbies like writing, playing the piano, Kung-fu, and many others, helped me stay productive during my quarantine. They have also helped me in my medical career by teaching me universal skills that have deepened my understanding of medical concepts (e.g., learning Kung-Fu helped me understand the actions of different muscles better). During the holidays, it is easy to become complacent, if you do not develop any skills outside of medicine. If you do not perform well in a test or exam, it can feel incredibly unfulfilling, especially if all you do is study for exams. Diversifying my skillset has become a useful safeguard for me during difficult times. I would have gone mad if I only studied during the quarantine.

11

PSYCHIATRY

Delving into patients' thoughts

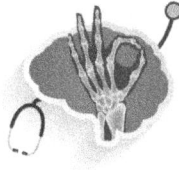

"Words of comfort, skillfully administered, are the oldest therapy known to man."

— *LOUIS NIZER*

The human brain is a fascinating organ that has incredible potential to change and adapt to new situations. Our ability to study all our undergraduate lectures in 4 weeks (shortened from 6 weeks as a result of the COVID-19 pandemic) is a testament to this. After my colleagues and I completed our 5th-year internal medicine block (which was mostly comprised of online Zoom lectures), we were summoned to the wards again, this time, at the mysterious Townhill Psychiatric Hospital.

Townhill Hospital seemed to be the perfect place for a Hollywood-style psychological thriller. The red face-brick hospital buildings with their looming spires and elegant British design seem to have been plucked straight out of a dark

Dickensian novel (Pietermaritzburg is renowned for its Victorian architecture). The sprawling hospital grounds were overgrown with weeds and bare trees that seemed to claw at the sky as if they were screaming in pain. Townhill exuded an idiosyncratic charm, that was intensified by the misty, hilly backdrop of Pietermaritzburg. A chill ran down my spine.

Pietermaritzburg was gripped in the icy throes of winter when I started my first psychiatry rotation. The hillside ward to which I was allocated was an unassuming lone building, surrounded by wire fences (to prevent certain patients from escaping) and ominous weeping willows. It was there where I formed the foundation of my understanding of psychiatry and its mysterious history and where I met my first psychiatric patient...who believed that he was a god.

I quickly realized that practicing psychiatry demands great patience, empathy, and skillful history taking. Our routine at Townhill hospital consisted of attending lectures and ward rounds with our consultants as well as clerking patients. Throughout my 4-week rotation, I was exposed to a cornucopia of fascinating patients and their concomitant mental conditions-psychotic disorders, anxiety disorders, depressive disorders...the list goes on.

The causes of many of these conditions are multifactorial. A person's genetics, childhood development, medical and social history are important determinants of mental health. Ergo, as part of our training, we were required to ask our patients many questions about these spheres of their lives, which allowed us intimate glimpses into their psyche.

MY FIRST PSYCHIATRY PATIENT

When I met my first psychiatry patient, Samuel (not his real name), he greeted me with a broad mischievous grin and an elbow bump (COVID-19 was still at large). I started my patient interview by asking him some general questions about his patient details, his main complaint, background history, and so forth...

He completely believed that he was the god of the moon and the reincarnation of the Last Airbender (a character from a popular TV show, which I enjoyed watching). Besides these so-called grandiose delusions, he had hardly slept for several days and felt an irresistible urge to chop as much wood as possible. This so-called manic episode caused his family to admit him to the psychiatric hospital. He often mentioned how he felt overwhelmed by pressure and judgment from his family and smoked cannabis to cope with stressors in his life.

I wondered: "what lead Samuel to think this way?" "What could have prevented this cascade of problems?" and, "what could psychiatric medicine do to help him?" The term, "psychiatry" is derived from the Greek words: psukhē ('soul, mind') and iatreia ('healing'-from iatros 'healer'). The term was first coined in 1808 by Reil, a professor of medicine in Germany. In his time, the predecessors of those we know as psychiatrists were known as," alienists" (those who treated mental alienation). This term was commonly used even until the twentieth century. Throughout the nineteenth century, confining patients with mental illnesses to, "therapeutic asylums" became the first-line measure of management. People with mental illnesses were being isolated from mainstream society both with words and physical barriers. Treatment options at the time were experimental and often inefficacious (e.g., purgatives, removal of teeth, enemas, bloodletting, and even gruesome frontal lobotomies). Vomiting was somehow believed to, "draw out" nervous irritants in the body. Around the 1930s the connection between evidence-based medicine and psychiatry took root. Now, our treatment armamentarium has expanded to include psychiatric drugs, psychotherapy (some of which are based on

Sigmund Freud's controversial psychosexual theories), electroconvulsive therapy (which involves inducing seizures in anesthetized patients), and other treatment modalities. The early history of psychiatry has been tumultuous. Many treatments have been unsuccessful and many mental illnesses are still not completely understood, even today (e.g., schizophrenia, which is one of the most common psychotic disorders). These many unknowns about mental health have helped breed uncertainty and fear in society. Horror movies, a thermometer of society's fears have often exploited this unnerving insecurity about the "other"-things we do not understand. Some people even express a macabre fascination with the "otherness" of mental health. The slasher genre of horror films is a testament to this fear of people with mental illnesses e.g., Jonathan Demme's The Silence of the Lambs (1991) and David Fincher's thriller Se7en (1995). Even now, one can find numerous serial killer documentaries on mainstream streaming platforms like Netflix. In some, however, fear breeds stigma.

This relegating of psychiatry to the shadows of medical science has persisted even until the 21st century. Despite this, mental health disorders have remained inextricably intertwined with shifts in society. The post-war period, dubbed "The Age of Anxiety" by W. H. Auden, was clouded by fears about the power of nuclear weapons, the Cold War arms race, and the possibility that communist spies were infiltrating society. This was a time when people were constantly watching or hearing news about capitalism versus communism. Many psychiatry patients of the time reported that they were being spied on by communists. My patient, Samuel, believed that he was being constantly watched by the "Suicide Squad"-characters from a DC comics superhero movie. We see pop culture characters very often in modern society. This delusion of persecution is the same as those noted in people during the Cold War, but the culture change has noticeably influenced the delusions. Interestingly, some cultures e.g., certain tribes in Africa and Asia see certain "psychotic symptoms" (e.g., hearing voices about ancestors) as gifts ordained by god. In my patient, Samuel, (who also believed that he could hear the voices of his ancestors) this is considered to be very abnormal in Western society.

Samuel was an incredibly pleasant individual who seemed to be quite intelligent (he graduated as a chemical engineer and was fond of mathematics). He performed well in school before he started to abuse marijuana and gradually developed psychotic and mood symptoms. He was responding well to treatment. I wondered about those who didn't. Talking to him was a fascinating experience. Our conversations seemed to bring him comfort as well. He often said that he felt like he had, "a lot to say", and was glad to meet somebody willing to listen. Despite the advances that we have made in psychiatry, a quote by Louis Nizer echoed in my mind: "Words of comfort, skillfully administered, are the oldest therapy known to man." I felt hopeful, knowing that his treatment and my listening helped him.

On my last day of clinical teaching at Townhill hospital, I returned to the hillside ward. While following an intern to help with a ward round, I got lost. On that day, the entire ward was stripped bare and the patients were shifted to another area in the hospital complex. There was nothing there besides the dusty linoleum floors, metal bedframes, and empty rooms. For a moment, I drank in the scene...the nothingness...the isolation. I imagined that Samuel and many other psychiatric patients over the ages must have felt that way when their illnesses set in and they were forced to face the double-edged sword of stigma and psychosis. I was overwhelmed with terror in that clinical labyrinth.

When I eventually found my way out of that barren ward, the sun shone through the overcast. From the hillside, I could see the whole hospital complex. I now associate that place with memories of helping others, who no longer seem like others, but ordinary people from my society, who just needed someone to talk to and the right treatments for their illnesses, like one needs a bandage for a cut. There were no horror movies or psychological thrillers there and the trees that surround the hospital now look as if they are searching for a helping hand.

Any medical student will tell you that medical school demands great mental fortitude. A 2017 systematic review and meta-analysis about mental health problems among medical students in brazil listed some common factors that contribute to mental health problems in medical students: A highly stressful environment, competitiveness, excessive workload, sleep deprivation, peer pressure, and many other personal, curricular, institutional, and affective factors. There are many more, but based on my discussions with many of my colleagues, these topics came up fairly frequently. These factors should not be underestimated and can cause conditions such as psychological stress, anxiety, depression, sleep pattern disorders, burnout, eating disorders, and potentially hazardous alcohol use in medical students. The list is much longer. Many suffer in silence. My class was hit hard in our 3rd year when we learned that one of our colleagues committed suicide. It was devastating news. I had spoken with her a few times. She was generally very pleasant and cheerful. Her passing hit us like a sledgehammer. We realized that it could happen to anyone.

Psychiatry is a fascinating subject that leads us to meet interesting people, with intriguing life stories. Some of them are filled with great suffering. One of my colleagues interviewed a psychotic patient who tried to stab himself through the heart but stabbed his lung instead. He survived, but the doctors believed that it was unlikely that he could ever live independently. It was a saddening thought and also a reminder that the patients we see daily can affect how we become as people. When one chooses to study a discipline in medicine, in addition to other important factors (e.g., time for family, compensation, intellectual stimulation) it is important to like the bread-and-butter cases-patients with conditions that you are likely to see daily.

Throughout medical school, I served as an executive member of the South African Medical Students Association (SAMSA). Eliminating the social stigma surrounding mental health problems and other conditions (e.g., TB) became a main theme for many of our community service campaigns. We started to realize how big a problem it was. People who wore N-95 masks in public were shunned (before the COVID-19 pandemic). Every day, we work to change this mindset. My advice to future medical students is to watch out for signs of common mental health conditions (e.g., depression-feelings of guilt/worthlessness, loss of interest and pleasure, changes in energy levels/sleeping habits/appetite/concentration, suicidal ideations...) in both yourselves and others. Seeking help early (e.g., from those who are close to you or from qualified healthcare providers), saves lives.

12

NEONATOLOGY

The smallest and cutest patients

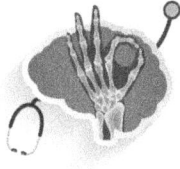

"A new baby is like the beginning of all things-wonder, hope, a dream of possibilities."

— *EDA J. LE SHAN*

Babies are very interesting patients. They can't tell you what is wrong with them. When they cry, it could mean anything. Is the baby hungry? Is the baby irritated? Is the baby feeling pain? We have to work that out ourselves through clinical examination and by asking the mothers questions. Following our psychiatry block (which is unofficially known as the most relaxed 5th-year block) we were thrust into a pressured 4-week clinical neonatology rotation in Edendale hospital, a short distance away from the Pietermaritzburg CBD. My brother and I rented out a 3-bedroom home in the verdant Victoria Country Club estate at the time (a last-minute stroke of luck). That meant daily 40-minute commutes (with traffic) to Edendale. Traffic gave us time to think and unwind. I loved downloading some of my favorite music and listening to top hit singles during those drives.

The road leading up to the hospital was dusty and constantly under construction. It was a subtle hint that resources would be limited in the hospital wards. Edendale hospital, one of the few regional hospitals in the area, was notorious for its high patient caseloads. We experienced it first-hand.

THE TRIALS AND TRIBULATIONS OF TINY PATIENTS

Every second day, we needed to report to the neonatal ward at 8:00 am to examine the newborns and take histories from their mothers (who usually breastfed their babies from 8:00 am onwards, at 3 hourly intervals). Owing to COVID-19 restrictions, we were not allowed to visit the hospital every day. I even got into trouble once for trying to examine patients in more than one ward. We desperately wanted to get as much clinical exposure as we could. Additionally, we were not permitted to enter the pediatric ward. It became apparent to us that clinical teaching would be limited to online case presentations and ward rounds, which were usually rushed to accommodate the daily waves of new patients. The doctors were pressed for time and often did not have much time to spare for students. As many medical students will tell you, acquiring signatures from doctors for our logbooks (a record of the work that we did) requires tact, good timing, and a bit of sweet-talking.

The first few days of a newborn's life are perilous. It was devastating to see so many children on ventilators. A condition known as respiratory distress syndrome was common amongst many of the newborns there. It is a condition in which fluid that lines the alveoli (the grape-like air sacs where gas exchange occurs in the lung) does not form properly, which leads to the collapse of the alveoli and breathing problems.

You have to be very careful when interacting with neonatal patients. During my pediatrics rotation in 4th year, I spent a few hours in the neonatal ward. There were just 2 patients. Both of them had a heart condition called a patent ductus arteriosus: a persistent opening between the two major blood vessels leading from the heart. In some patients, it doesn't cause a problem. If it is very large, it can be problematic for the neonates. Trying to open the incubator, examine the neonate and position my stethoscope to hear the famous machinery murmur (an abnormal heart sound that can be heard in patients with a PDA) without waking the baby, feels like a Mission Impossible heist scene. Some babies can be so irritable that they won't allow you to examine them, without crying excessively. During my 5th year, I examined a baby with an arched back and a very abnormal posture (called opisthotonos). She also had several cardiac defects and a history of recurrent infections. She stayed in the same ward for almost the whole 3 weeks of our neonatology rotation. Whenever we tried to examine her, she woke up and screamed for minutes on end. She could not be appeased. She usually cried herself back to sleep. It was heart-breaking. Another baby was less than 1kg in weight. She could fit inside the palm of my hand. For weeks, she suffered from cardiac defects and was given oxygen. Her skin was blue, because not enough oxygen was getting into her bloodstream. I felt helpless. I could only trust the decisions of the senior doctors.

What astounded me was the resilience of the neonates. They are a prime example of life's willingness to persevere, despite immense odds. After a few days of treatment, many of the children were healthy enough to be transferred to the less intensive Kangaroo Mother care ward, where the mothers could spend time with their children after they stabilized. There, they could cuddle with their babies and learn how to breastfeed and care for them optimally.

Neonates want to be held. Physical contact is incredibly important for a baby's survival. When you touch a neonate for the first time, to examine him/her, you first notice how incredibly soft their skin is. Their bodies can fit inside both of your hands. Neonates have a reflex where if you place something like a finger onto their palm, they naturally hold onto it, by curling their fingers around it. It just melts the heart. Neonates draw out paternal or maternal instincts that you never thought you had. One feels instinctively compelled to protect them. The neonates have an instinct to hold on-to survive.

Seeing a neonate recover is incredibly rewarding, especially for the anxious mothers who constantly worry about the wellbeing of their children. They are incredibly delicate and endure probably the hardest phase of their lives during their first few days after birth. We must help them through it as best as we can. After all, they will replace all of us.

The neonates reminded me of myself when I first started medical school. Much like them, we faced a challenging series of trials and tribulations to grow and develop in a new environment. We had to learn critical new skills and attain new developmental milestones. We wrote our first medical theory test. We learned how to use a stethoscope and a dissecting kit for the first time. We learned how to do basic CPR. Of course, attaining milestones in childhood or medical school should be achieved within certain timeframes. Some learn faster than others. Some take longer. Accepting this is important as well. Some of your colleagues may be better than you in some areas. It is important to learn from those who perform better than you and to help those who may be having trouble achieving those milestones. I, for example, had trouble intubating a CPR dummy, for the first time in 3rd year. I eventually mastered it in 5th year, during my emergency medicine skills training, after multiple practice attempts. Once, I didn't remove an IV needle correctly from a patient. Her blood spurted from her wound, like a hose. Parents tend to become concerned when their children don't achieve their milestones within specific timeframes. I felt the same way when I felt that I did not master a clinical skill within a set time. Often, these time frames have a certain degree of flexibility. You might not be able to master auscultation (e.g., listening for heart sounds) immediately in 2nd year. It takes time and practice. But, if you keep at it, you will get there. That is an important lesson that I also learned from my Kung Fu practice. Kung Fu essentially translates to: "Time and Practice." An important Kung Fu philosophy is that there can be no transformation without hardship-pushing ourselves beyond our limits.

Many believe that there are higher levels of Maslow's hierarchy of needs-beyond self-actualization. One of these higher-order tiers is self-transcendence: "The ability of human beings to find meaning by being directed toward something or someone, other than themselves" Some studies suggest that focusing on improving the lives of others results in better work engagement among nurses and possibly other healthcare professionals. I strongly support this concept. The idea of, "paying it forward" to help your colleagues goes a long way. When we are all in the neonatal phases of our medical careers, supporting each other helps immensely, especially if that support comes from more senior people. In the Kangaroo Mother Care ward at Edendale hospital, an important philosophy in the ward is: "Mothers help mothers." The ward was essentially a series of cozy interconnected rooms with closely spaced beds, where mothers and their newborns could rest and huddle up together. Many of the mothers I spoke to did not know how to breastfeed or help their ailing children. The mothers supported each other. The more experienced mothers taught the new mothers valuable advice about breastfeeding techniques, even if they hardly knew each other. It was a comforting testament to human camaraderie and it reminded me of my experiences in the obstetrics and gynecology ward at Mahatma Gandhi Hospital 1 year before.

I promoted self-transcendence in our medical school, by starting a student-led lecturing society, which I called BROCA (named after a part of the brain which co-ordinates voluntary speech). My brother and I recruited some other passionate medical students from our year to teach younger students critical lessons about public speaking and other medical subjects. We are very passionate about speaking and writing. I realized that speaking forms a crucial part of our experience with patients as well as our oral exams. So, we decided to use BROCA to educate others about the importance of this and to help them with their studies. We also designed practice assessments for the younger students. Most of our presentations were met with large crowds of students and for a while, we were the most active student organization on campus. Many of the students were fond of our passionate high-energy presentations-a stark contrast to many other lecturers who merely read from PowerPoint presentations. It was a great deal of fun helping the other students attain their medical developmental milestones faster, by sharing our experiences and knowledge. It was also an opportunity for us to revise our basic medical knowledge. Eventually, when we graduated from the school of laboratory medicine, we could not be on campus frequently. Since then, BROCA started to place greater emphasis on communication through writing, which was an opportunity for me to explore my interest in medical writing.

Helping others led me to unexpected situations in medical school, which I welcomed wholeheartedly. While surfing the internet, I came across a website for Habitat for Humanity-an NGO that aims to construct homes in underdeveloped communities. I thought that this was an amazing opportunity to help others and learn a new skill-construction. I sent them an e-mail asking if I could also educate people about HIV and TB, during the construction project, while helping with the building process (another example of how asking for help can yield great opportunities). They agreed willingly.

During the building days, I met some incredible people from prominent businesses in and around Durban. The project took place in a small rural community on the South Coast called Umgababa, where community leaders still make the final decisions concerning the people of Umgababa. It was a long 45-minute drive along the N2, but it was a refreshing chance to enjoy the beautiful views of Durban's south coast. The air is fresh there. On one side of the road, you see the sparkling Indian Ocean. On the other, you can see rolling hills. I got lost a few times, but eventually, I made it to the small Umgababa community. Imagine winding dirt roads, flocks of chickens, small spaza shops with Coca-Cola advertisements, and small settlements scattered across the hills. When we received approval from the community leaders, we started building after a few weeks. I helped set up an HIV testing tent, with help from the university and brought in a few of my friends from the medical school to help start building the foundation for one of the homes. It was great fun, despite the heavy labor. We helped clear a lot of the debris from the construction sites. I will never forget the small moments like sharing a cold beverage with our friends from ABSA (Amalgamated Banks of South Africa) or joining in prayer with the recipients of one of the homes that we helped construct. Helping others helps us in unexpected ways and it has helped me attain my medical developmental milestones faster and more effectively-especially in terms of improving my communication skills.

During the early years of our life, as well as in medical school we make many mistakes. This is natural. I, myself tried many strategies to improve my studying technique. Even now, I am still constantly refining it, to find a strategy that best works for me. When I started medical school, I was frustrated. I felt that I was not performing as well as I did in high school. Medicine is a different ball game entirely. Old strategies might not always suffice. Hard work, discipline, and perseverance is required, regardless of the situation.

Dr. Brian Goldman, an emergency-room physician in Toronto made a compelling TED talk about the topic of doctors making mistakes. There is this prevailing culture of perfectionism in medicine. Everybody assumes that doctors are infallible beings with the ability to heal almost anything. Any doctor who makes a mistake-like administering an incorrect drug dosage (which is more common than you would expect) is met with awkward silences and an onslaught from the media. Granted, there is a certain degree of skill that is expected from physicians with a certain level of training, but one must take into account human error. Dr. Goldman argues that we must talk about our errors to promote a culture of learning and health promotion, rather than hide our errors and risk further harm to future patients. I saw this myself. At Inkosi Albert Luthuli Central Hospital I attended a grand round in the neurology ward. It was both an intimidating and inspiring experience. The most skilled neurologists in the province gathered together for the round to discuss and present the patients. They were incredibly knowledgeable. I recognized some of them who wrote chapters in our textbooks. They barely paid any attention to me or the other students, while we stared at them in awe. The head neurologist asked one of the registrars a question about Parkinson disease (a disorder of the central nervous system that affects movement, often including tremors). His answer didn't satisfy. The registrar was met with a headshake of disapproval from the head neurologist and awkward silence from the rest of the doctors.

Eventually, when the ward round was done, the doctors left for an MRI meeting. An MRI uses powerful magnets to help form highly detailed images of the human body. It is very useful for looking for masses in the spinal cord. The other students had left, but I was curious. I wanted to know what they discussed behind closed doors. I was wearing a suit at the time, so I guess that the neurologists assumed that I was another registrar or intern. I snuck into the room. I must admit that I was genuinely surprised.

We looked at several MRIs and the neurologists couldn't come up with a single diagnosis. Granted, more tests could have been done, but my entire view of the quintessential singular master physician shifted. Even when all of them worked together, they didn't come up with a single diagnosis. There was no flash of revelatory diagnostic wizardry. It was a series of: "It could be this or I might be mistaken." It was a matter of sifting out the most probable provisional diagnosis from a list of very similar differential diagnoses. There was a clear hierarchy. The doctor's feared making mistakes in front of the superiors. But the superiors were allowed to make mistakes without fear of reprisal. This was not the first time that I had witnessed this.

During my anesthetics rotation in my 4th year, I observed an orthopedic operation on an elderly woman. I had attended several surgeries before with one of the specialist anesthetists. He tried to inject a spinal anesthetic which was somewhat challenging because the woman was overweight. He must have tried at least 12 times. I have noticed many occasions where even experts make mistakes. Talking about these kinds of errors allows us to help each other. By reflecting on them, we realize our shortcomings, help future patients and help other members of the healthcare team achieve and master their medical developmental milestones.

I often thought about this during the neonatology block. When we start going to university and living independently, we achieve a big milestone. We enter the world of adulthood and leave the safety of childhood. Adulthood and childhood come with different challenges and different joys, but both do not have to be mutually exclusive. We were all neonates once…even the seemingly mean consultants who berate us. There were times when we were all vulnerable, when we made mistakes and when we needed someone to hold. Even as adults, we need that sometimes. I feel that our inner neonate represents that part of our more vulnerable selves that needs protection from challenges in adulthood. We can make it easier by being there for each other like the KMC mothers. We must keep holding on.

13

OBSTETRICS

Rebirth of a system

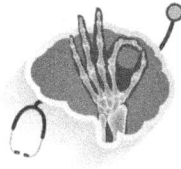

"In giving birth to our babies, we may find that we give birth to new possibilities within ourselves."

— *MYLA KABAT-ZINN*

S tarting anything new in medical school feels like a rebirth of ourselves. When we move from one discipline to the next, our way of thinking usually has to change a lot. It was around early November 2020, when I started my obstetrics block. By then, life was moving like clockwork. Each day flowed into the other in a predictable routine. The days became a cycle of 3-week blocks followed by 1 week of exams. The method of examination had to change to ensure that social distancing was maintained. Most of our exams were changed from in-person assessments to online assessments involving paper patient cases. Essentially, we were required to read a story about a patient on a sheet of paper and discuss that patient with our examiner, who was on the other side of a computer screen. Zoom was the app of choice for our clinical tutorials and exams.

We were examined in 3 ways in medical school. Theory exams (written multiple-choice questions), OSCEs (objectively structured clinical exams in which we were required to examine patients and suggest a plan for managing them), and portfolio exams (which involved discussing one of our case reports with a doctor).

My father studied at UKZN. Many of his lecturers and examiners were still working full-time at the university during my medical school years. During my 4th-year internal medicine exam, I was graded by the same doctor who examined my dad for his final year assessments. I joked about this with her, before she assessed me-to her great amusement.

Our university feels monolithic in the way that it approaches medical teaching. Not much has changed in terms of the style of teaching. But gradually, transformation is becoming more noticeable. UKZN has seen its fair share of student protests and financial problems, but things are still improving. In its glory days, UKZN medical school was known as the best medical school in the country. Even now the standards are very high. Students must excel in high school before they can even be considered for acceptance. Many of the doctors have mixed opinions about the state of our medical school. Some feel that there has been a slow deterioration in the quality of medical teaching. Others report that we are still at the top of our game. I believe that the quality of graduating medical doctors is mostly dependent on the willingness of the individual medical students to engage with their material and that the onus should not be solely placed on the teaching clinicians. The responsibility is largely on us. I think that if you work hard, you will likely excel, regardless of the quality of your medical school teaching. Irrespective of the way everything operated in the past, things needed to change drastically, in response to the COVID-19 pandemic. It was a rebirth of the system.

REBIRTH AND REPRODUCTION

Birth is one of the most dangerous and rewarding times in a woman's life. Both pregnancy and delivery put the mother and fetus at risk of potentially life-threatening conditions like sepsis, intrauterine fetal death (where the baby dies in the womb), and hemorrhage. Bhagwan Shree Rajneesh stated: "The moment a child is born, the mother is also born. She never existed before. The woman existed, but the mother, never. A mother is something absolutely new." Many women report a feeling of indescribable joy when they become mothers. It was a soul-stirring moment that I had the privilege of witnessing in the Edendale hospital labor ward.

Owing to COVID-19 restrictions, we could only spend 2 days in the labor ward (one of which was a night call from 4:00 pm to 10:00 pm). Our obstetrics rotation lasted 3 weeks. 1 week was spent learning the online resources. The other 2 weeks were spent either in the maternity ward or in the obstetrics ward. My brother quipped that we were learning medicine in reverse-after having studied pediatrics the week before.

We quickly learned that there were a few medical conditions that we had to learn very well for obstetrics (e.g., hypertension/high blood pressure, diabetes, eclampsia-where the blood vessels in the placenta develop abnormally, miscarriages, and a few others). Precision, timing, and measurements were important aspects of learning obstetrics. In our exam, we were asked many questions about the measurement of the pelvis and the different trimesters of pregnancy.

Modern obstetrics has come a long way since the childbirth practices of ancient civilizations. To put things into perspective, The Egyptians believed that the uterus, "wandered about the abdomen like an animal in response to odors or to engulf a man's seed during coitus." They also believed that a woman could become pregnant after oral sex. Now there are numerous textbooks covering topics ranging from contraception to childbirth, in great detail, down to the molecular level.

Even the devices used to aid delivery have evolved drastically (even if some still resemble medieval torture machines)- (google "a weighted Auvard speculum"). The Hebrews used bamboo shoots during the 1300s as an early version of the modern speculum.

During our gynecology rotation in my 4th year, we were required to visit a clinic known as the Commercial City Clinic in the Durban CBD. The university bus dropped us off on the streets outside the clinic, wide-eyed and slightly lost, with only our lab coats to distinguish us from the morass of Durbanites and foreigners from neighboring African countries who were selling their wares on the streets. I remember that day vividly. It felt as if I was walking through hot and bustling downtown New Delhi. We spent the rest of that scorching day learning about and administering various forms of contraception and protection to female patients at the clinic, from condoms to pills and intrauterine copper devices. Owing to the prevalence of HIV in our country, family planning remains an especially important way to help prevent the further spread of the virus.

Along with contraception, we were briefly exposed to Caesarean deliveries in the operating room at Mahatma Gandhi Memorial Hospital. During my 5th year, I helped with my first vaginal delivery. It was a profound experience.

My brother and I were examining patients in the labor ward at Edendale hospital. It was an uncomfortably warm and compact space, filled with patient beds. There was little space for much else. A fierce tempest raged on outside. The ward was intermittently shaken by the sound of intense thunder. It was late at night and the downpour outside came unexpectedly.

Screams are not uncommon in the labor ward. The nurses there have become inured to it. I imagine that this attitude is the product of years of experience working in that high-pressure environment. It was still a bit jarring for me. The screams are jarring and are to be expected from many women during childbirth-which is, reportedly, one of the greatest physical pains any human can experience.

One of the nurses asked us to assist with a vaginal delivery. I felt my pulse quicken from excitement and urgency. This was my first time seeing a vaginal delivery and I wanted to help as much as I could. Many medical students also see aiding childbirth as a rite of passage. Delivering babies is an ancient practice that has been refined over countless generations. The woman was slightly overweight and in her 30s. We were concerned that it would be a difficult delivery. Nonetheless, the nurse's hands moved deftly. She administered the oxytocin at the right time (a drug that helps the uterus push out the baby) and advised the mother to push hard. My brother and I offered the mother our support and helped provide the nurse with the equipment that she needed. The mother's face was drenched in sweat. She breathed at an increasingly faster pace. We could just see the baby's head. "Push!" we all shouted in unison.

And just like that, a new life was brought into the world.

The baby was put to the mother's breast immediately. She breathed an overwhelming sigh of relief. "Is it a boy or a girl?" she panted. "A girl!" the nurse shouted cheerfully. The mother's eyes widened. Then she smiled in a way that I will never forget. It was an expression of a pure, uninhibited joy-a smile of renewal that lit up her face. At that moment, I understood what Bhagwan Shree Rajneesh meant. The woman seemed instantaneously younger in the moment of her smile. The moment happened so quickly, sans the quintessential

Hollywood-style flair and dramatic crying. It was a subtle, quiet joy.

I reflected on that moment when my brother and I drove home through the dark valleys of Pietermaritzburg around 10:00pm.

That child was born into an incredibly tumultuous time in the history of humanity. The storm could be a metaphor for that. The COVID-19 pandemic drastically changed how we lived. That girl was born into a time when her family could not touch her in the way that they could, one year before.

I chose to see the pandemic as a rebirth in the way that we approach things. Old systems that did not place enough emphasis on good hygiene (which is still the most effective medical intervention known to humans) were shown to be flawed and unsustainable. Professor Siddhartha Mukherjee once wrote: "There's a glassy transparency to things around us that work, made visible only when the glass is cracked and fissured. Look, it's nothing. To dwell inside a well-functioning machine is to be largely unaware of its functioning. That's its gift, and we accept it thoughtlessly, ungratefully, unknowingly." The pandemic was just another crucible that forced us to renew our approaches to many things in life…even if the costs were devastating.

I wrote this article on Christmas eve, which for many is a festive time. It is a time of rebirth for many-which for me was a recurring theme in 2020. By that time, COVID-19 vaccines were being distributed in several countries across the world. The news brought hope. The news was an island of joy surrounded by a raging tempest, much like the child we helped deliver.

The screams of the women in the labor ward were the product of the immense pain of delivery…but that pain was the prerequisite to overwhelming happiness that many of those women experienced when they saw their children for the first time.

COVID-19 brought much death and pain, but it showed us where things needed to change and where we needed to change. I learned to appreciate time with my family more. Simple things matter a lot more to me now, especially because they were briefly taken away by COVID-19. I missed walks along the beach, the feeling of a cool breeze against my face, and firmly shaking the hand of a good friend.

Adapting to external stressors is essential for healthcare and humanity. It is deeply entrenched in our biology-much like how the female pelvis has changed in response to our longer lifespans and new methods of delivery. The COVID-19 pandemic was just another of those stressors. Like childbirth or any other challenge, there will be suffering, but the reward, in this case, is a safer world where the little girl, who we helped deliver, can one day hug her family without fear.

COMMUNITY HEALTH

Back to basics

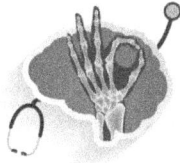

"Success is all about consistency around the fundamentals."

— *ROBIN SHARMA*

W e had to go back to basics. Primary health care was our final clinical rotation for 2020. Many interns argue that primary healthcare is the most important subject to learn for the daily practical application of our medical knowledge. During the block, we learned valuable skills like how to run a private practice and how to report and manage problematic situations in a medical facility (called adverse events). Much of the block was dedicated to teaching us these practical skills, which kept us grounded in a clinic setting. Too often, working in public healthcare facilities feels like street-fighting medicine (a combat zone where you survive by doing what works, even if it is unconventional). I have seen some doctors pocket blood tubes so that they will have a backup stash if stock runs out in the wards. I was reminded of the doctor from Prince Mshiyeni who used a skateboard to travel between the wards faster. Owing to the large patient caseloads that healthcare professionals see daily, in a primary healthcare setting, many of us have come up with some creative solutions.

It's no wonder that social media accounts and books with names like:" Intern survival guide" have been created by some doctors to help us navigate through the landscape of primary healthcare. It feels like a battleground and you're the outnumbered commander.

In my 4th year, during one night call at Prince Mshiyeni hospital, there was only one doctor available. Besides me, there was one other 6th-year student and 2 nurses. That was our entire team. We had to last the night and manage patients in the emergency room and the medical wards, which were quite far apart. I can understand why some doctors feel strained by their workload. Some of them even work for 24-hour shifts and longer, in some hospitals, which is a significant contributor to physician burnout-a long-term stress reaction marked by emotional exhaustion, depersonalization, and a lack of sense of personal accomplishment.

There is one important thing to clarify. Based on what I have seen in medical school, medicine is not all glamour. Yes, it is a beautiful and highly fulfilling profession-emotionally, psychologically, spiritually, and financially. But it is demanding as well. Many 1st year students start the degree with the assumption that medicine will be like Grey's Anatomy-stylish and well-groomed doctors in well-equipped facilities using astounding diagnostic skills to manage complex medical cases.

Yes, you may experience that and it is part of what makes medicine fun and exciting. But much of your time during your years as a student may be spent dealing with common primary healthcare problems like high blood pressure, diabetes, TB, and HIV, which require you to follow constantly changing guidelines. I emphasize that it is important to enjoy the bread-and-butter cases-patients with conditions that you will see almost every day. Of course, for many, enthusiasm starts to wane, once you've seen your 100th diabetes case. Taking the time to master the basics well, will go a long way to helping you in a primary healthcare setting. Many of our consultants are fond of this quote:" Common things occur commonly." The phrase:" Zebra" is heard in some American medical schools. It is American medical slang for arriving at a surprising, often exotic, medical diagnosis when a more commonplace explanation is more likely. It comes from an old saying used in teaching medical students about how to think logically about differential diagnosis: "When you hear hoofbeats, think of horses, not zebras". Interestingly enough, there were several actual zebras that lived outside our home in Pietermaritzburg. I admit that I fell into this trap in 1st year. It feels fun to diagnose a patient with a rare disease, but you must consider the most likely conditions first. You will learn to come up with a broad list of possible differential diagnoses (what condition you think the patient may have), most of which are common things that you will see in primary healthcare. Thinking broadly is important in clinical medicine.

Part of primary healthcare is family medicine, where we learn a lot of other important disciplines of medicine that aren't normally seen elsewhere in other subjects. Some of these disciplines include sexual medicine, travel medicine, palliative care medicine, and communication skills. These are still incredibly important subjects to learn and we were given many assignments to ensure that we understood them well (even if they left us a bit exhausted at the end of the year).

I recall taking a sexual history from a male patient. I realized then the importance of understanding my patients' cultures, especially when asking them intimate and personal questions. Eliciting the patient's sexual history required sensitivity and tact. He initially refused to explain his sexual problems to me in the presence of his mother and another female chaperone. He helped me realize the importance of erectile function as a symbol of masculinity and confidence amongst many South African men. He also explained to me that this was the reason why he felt inadequate and ashamed about addressing his sexual problems when they first started. Talking to the patient man-to-man and reassuring him that problems with erectile function and sexual satisfaction are common, helped me build rapport with him and obtain a more detailed sexual history. The patient also helped me realize the importance of differentiating between organic causes (e.g., diabetes) and psychosexual causes (e.g., stressful job, performance anxiety) of erectile dysfunction and the need to address both concurrently. Speaking to the patient helped me think about the importance of educating both the patient and his partner about erectile dysfunction and involving both of them in future counseling sessions, to ensure that they worked together to alleviate the psychosexual determinants of their sexual and relationship problems. Expect to get personal with your patients. Be ready to talk about anything which can range from topics about foods that they like to what their sex life is like.

It was a very sensitive topic of discussion. Medicine forces us to look inwards and address our fears. We are often pushed beyond our comfort zones. I remember my first visit to our anatomy dissecting hall in 1st year. One of my colleagues fainted, when she saw a dead body for the first time. Now, seeing dead bodies and signing death certificates at the end of a long night in the emergency room is commonplace. We have become desensitized to it. Even taking blood tends to make many people squeamish. We are forced to overcome things that discomfort us, in our profession. Most people don't think that they can last more than 24 hours without sleep, before they study medicine. Medicine pushes you beyond your limits in that way…and changes our approaches to death and dying.

Palliative care is another important subject that we were required to learn for our primary healthcare block. Palliative care is generally offered to a patient when curative treatment is no longer viable. This type of care is focused on providing relief from the symptoms and stress of the illness. The goal is to improve the quality of life for both the patient and the family. This discipline tends to make some doctors feel uncomfortable. It compels us to accept that we do not have a panacea. Sometimes, people can't handle telling others that they won't make it. Sometimes, we can't cure patients. For many healthcare professionals, this is difficult to accept. Some see an inability to cure as a failure of medical science. We indeed have a long way to go and we must constantly improve our understanding of medicine e.g., through research. However, it is important to remember that an important aspect of medicine is the ethical principle of beneficence and non-maleficence (we must do what is in the best interest of the patient and we must do no harm to the patient). In our medical school exams, clinicians are fond of asking us profound ethical questions based on clinical scenarios. Here is one profound example: There is a pair of conjoined twins who need a life-saving operation. If the operation is not done, both will die. If the operation is done, you can only save one. Which one will you save? Medicine does that to you. It challenges your own biases and insecurities and pushes you towards making evidence-based decisions for the betterment of humanity. Some of your views will be challenged. Some people support women's rights to abort a fetus. Some don't. What will you do when a patient comes to you to request one? You have to put the patient's needs before your own or at least refer them to someone who will if it is not in line with your values. The Hippocratic oath demands that all doctors do this.

During my primary healthcare block, I was required to take a detailed history from a patient with lung cancer and discuss the possibility of death with her. It was not an easy conversation to have.

She felt that she was gradually coming to terms with her illness and often read magazines and books about cancer that were provided by her local hospice. She expected the hospice and hospital teams to help her manage her pain and continue to supply her with more educational resources to help her learn more about cancer e.g., magazines and books. She felt deeply saddened by the thought that she didn't have much time left. This was coupled with her fear of infection by COVID-19. She wanted to spend more time with her sister and her neighbors, in her final days, as she missed them dearly when she was in the hospital. She was alone in the hospital. Her friends and family did not visit the hospital often as they, too, feared COVID-19 infection. She requested a do-not-resuscitate advanced directive (which meant that she did not want anyone to try to resuscitate her in the final moments of her life). She wanted to pass away peacefully. She considered herself to be more spiritual than religious and found that daily prayer offered her comfort, meaning, and opportunities to reflect on her illness and the importance of her sister. She wished for more time to pray and reflect and wished for the medical team and the hospice team to offer her a quiet place to pray in the morning.

Understanding people's needs during the final hours of their lives tends to shift our priorities. It is a reminder that we should appreciate the importance of staying healthy and spending time with the people who matter to us. As I wrote this, COVID-19 continued to claim hundreds of thousands of lives across the globe. Every day, I received messages from friends and family who were infected. Some were on ventilators. Some didn't make it. Almost every hospital bed for COVID-19 patients in my city was occupied. Some of my intern friends were signing death certificates every day, for COVID-19 patients. On some days, elective surgeries could not be done, because the oxygen pressure to ventilate surgical patients in the operating theatres was too low. The demand for oxygen in the COVID wards was just too high…

Despite the turmoil that gripped our society, we still needed to complete our studies. For our primary healthcare block, our schedule worked like this: We were expected to visit Northdale hospital in Pietermaritzburg every alternate day. During the days when we were at home, we were advised to learn the online resources that were provided to us and attend online tutorials using Zoom as a platform.

During the 3-week block, we were also required to complete a series of assignments and reflections about various family medicine disciplines (e.g., travel medicine, palliative care, management of a private practice, how to manage adverse events, emergency medicine, and sexual medicine). It was our final push for the year. Some disciplines in medical school require you to complete a lot of assignments and personal reflections.

Northdale hospital is another regional hospital in Pietermaritzburg. The hospital complex is arranged in tiers along a hilly terrain. That design led to a hilarious encounter between me and one of the hospital staff. Both I and a colleague assumed that the only way to move between the hospital tiers was to climb up the rusty ladders that connected one tier to the other. The hospital staff shot confused looks at us as we climbed. I had to catch my colleague once when he almost fell of the ladder. It almost collapsed under our weight. Eventually, one of the security guards slowly walked up to us and directed us to a nearby staircase. In our defense…the stairs were hard to find.

Our first week was spent in the ARV (antiretroviral) clinic. South Africa has some of the highest numbers of people living with HIV/AIDS in the world. ARVs are drugs that help decrease the replication of HIV in the body, which helps patients with

HIV/AIDS manage their condition. Fortunately, CAPRISA operates right next to our university. It serves as a global leader in HIV/AIDS research. Our time in the ARV clinic was an important opportunity to learn more about one of the most common bread-and-butter conditions that we will see in practice. On our first day, we were a bit late, as we couldn't find the place (the ARV clinic was on the highest tier of the hospital complex). A colleague and I were assigned to a doctor who was doing his year of community service (at the time that I wrote this, all medical school graduates were required to complete 2 years of internship at a public hospital, followed by one year of community service). He was a great teacher, who took the time to educate us about the ARV regimens in his spare time (which was often limited). Teaching isn't the main priority for many of the doctors. We were lucky if they spared a moment to teach us.

Most of the time, we sat in the clinic with the doctor and listened in on consultations with patients living with HIV/AIDS. Owing to the high patient caseloads, consultations were usually brief and involved asking the patients rapid-fire questions based on a series of checklists such as: "Are you taking your medication?" or, "Do you know your viral load?" Most consultations only lasted about 5 minutes. Ideally, we wanted to spend as much time with the patients as possible, but as most doctors will tell you: "You need to push the queue if. You want to finish on time."

For primary healthcare, we needed to learn many guidelines, inside-out. We needed to know which ARVs to give to the patient and when. We needed to know all the side effects of the different drug classes. We needed to know how the drugs interacted with each other. We needed to do this for tuberculosis, hypertension, and diabetes guidelines as well (along with a few others). It was a lot to learn in 3 weeks. Fortunately, the South African government helped us out and designed an app for quickly accessing all of this information (which is an invaluable tool, according to many of my friends who are doing their internship).

For a whole week, we took histories and examined patients, in the ARV clinic. We came to the worrying realization that a large portion of our patients were young people in their teens or 20s. The head of the ARV clinic was a genial doctor who hosted a weekly youth clinic day-a day where young people living with HIV/AIDS could talk to each other and healthcare professionals about living with their disease.

During the youth clinic day, we dispelled some myths and allayed fears (many people don't know that HIV is mainly transmitted through sexual intercourse or blood products). But that was only a small group of patients. There are millions more out there, but at least it was a start for us. Many of the younger children looked confused and withdrawn (as if they did not know why they were there). Many were younger than 16 years of age. One of the older children took charge of the discussion when the other healthcare professionals left (Lord-of-the-Flies style). He was energetic and spoke extensively about marijuana, his desire for sex, and whether he would be given food for the next youth clinic day. His speech was a strong reminder that HIV/AIDS is largely determined by social factors. Managing diseases is rarely ever just the responsibility of the government. Society needs to work together to manage them effectively. Our time in the ARV clinic drove that idea home for us. In light of the COVID-19 pandemic and our time in the ARV clinic, I could not help but reflect on viruses-including the human papillomavirus, which I researched during the first 2 years of my research placement at CAPRISA. Through my research, I learned a lot about how clinical studies are designed, how cells send signals to each other, and why it is so important for us to prevent viruses from spreading-e.g., through interventions like vaccinations.

MY FIRST MEDICAL RESEARCH ASSIGNMENT

I think we owe a lot to viruses…there, I said it.

David J. Griffiths' study on retroviruses further supports the evidence that at least 8% of the human genome is derived from retroviruses. They became integrated into our DNA millions of years ago, to replicate better and are essentially a part of us. They have been around for longer than us and they will probably be around long after we are gone. These human endogenous retroviruses (or HERVs) have some important functions, such as aiding the formation of the human placenta. Alas… some retroviruses would sooner kill you than help you reproduce. And I have had the pleasure of studying them intimately.

HIV (Human Immunodeficiency Virus) is ubiquitous in clinical settings, throughout KwaZulu Natal. In KZN; HIV is notorious and highly feared (it can be transmitted through needle stick injuries, through sexual contact and through giving birth). HIV is morbidly elegant. One cannot help but admire how it infects us; in the way that one would admire a tactfully executed bank heist. HIV binds to receptors on our immune cells (like the CD4 molecule on T-helper cells, which help co-ordinate other cells in our immune system, or the CCR5 and CXCR4 receptors on macrophages-which are important cells that eat and present foreign molecules to our immune systems).

I have learned much about this devastating virus during lectures, my hospital rounds and as part of my research with my mentor at CAPRISA: Dr. Lenine Liebenberg (who is amazing and always offers me coffee, during our meetings).

She asked me to look into another virus-Human Papilloma Virus (HPV)-which has been a research interest of mine for some time. Studying HPV improved my research skills greatly.

HPV is the main culprit behind almost all kinds of cervical cancer-the cancer that affected the young aspiring film star I examined in the Mahatma Gandhi gynecology ward. HPV can hijack the replication machinery of epithelial cells and make viral proteins, which can disrupt the epithelial cell growth cycle (and can cause cancers). There are many types of HPV. HPV types 16 and 18 cause over 70% of cervical cancer cases and can be prevented with vaccines e.g., Gardasil. Many governments around the world have been trying to make these vaccines available to the young children who need them.

Aah! So, both HIV and HPV can use our machinery against us. Now, Dr. Liebenberg posed this question to me, "How does HPV affect one's risk of getting HIV?"-What will happen when two masters of the heist join forces? The study was underway...

779 women were enrolled in the CAPRISA 004 study, to evaluate how well tenofovir 1% gel (an antiretroviral drug/ARV that helps slow down the replication of HIV) would work in preventing HIV infection. The trial was completed in 2010. Specimens were collected from these women in the form of cervicovaginal lavage (basically, you inject 3ml of saline water into a woman's ectocervix and aspirate the liquid that comes out). The liquid was centrifuged (spun at really high speeds) to form a pellet from which HPV DNA was extracted. HPV is another sexually transmitted virus that can cause genital warts and cervical cancer. These pellets were tested for organisms that cause sexually transmitted infections, concentrations of tenofovir, and cytokines (which are chemical signals that allow cells to communicate with each other).

Now, like many of my colleagues; I have heard the word, "cytokines" ad infinitum. It is easy to be confused by the sheer number of different cytokines, many of which have very different roles, within the body. They are substances (e.g., proteins) that are released by cells and have a specific effect on the interactions and communications between cells-they are signals, which help cells talk to each other and guide each other. Dr. Lenine Liebenberg and her team measured these chemical signals in the pellets. Some interesting results were elucidated...

HPV causes inflammation in the female reproductive system. The HPV infected cells say, "Wait just a minute here! There is an invader in our midst." They release the cytokines/chemical signals to attract white blood cells/ defenders of the body, like T helper cells and other immune cells...a distress signal.

But an ambush has been set...

This inflammatory response may clear a person of HPV (clearance). However, people can still maintain their HPV (persist) or even gain new HPV types (acquired). Dr. Liebenberg's study showed that clearance is linked to the biggest differences in cytokine levels and that cytokine levels are increased in women who have HPV compared to women without HPV (especially certain cytokines that are linked to HIV risk).

The immune cells arrive at the cervical epithelium, prepared for combat with HPV. But, the trap springs! HIV, lying in wait, infects the reinforcements-a ploy worthy of Sun Tzu's approval.

The results of the study showed that through such a tactic; HPV can increase a woman's risk of acquiring HIV several times more than if she were HPV negative (especially if the woman's immune system is robust enough to recruit more immune cells to the cervix). This risk is even higher for women with oncogenic/high-risk cancer-causing HPV types. Understanding that deepened my understanding of the disease that caused so much suffering for the young aspiring film star in the gynecology ward. If I shared that knowledge with her, maybe it could have helped her understand her disease better.

The study highlights the importance of preventing HPV infection in our population, where HPV and HIV are prevalent. The rollout of new HPV vaccines in South African schools has the potential to further help prevent the spread of both HPV and HIV, by disrupting their sinister synergy. Maybe if we started the vaccine rollout earlier, we could have saved the patient in Mahatma Ghandi hospital. Maybe she would have lived long enough to become a famous film star. Educating our population about the importance of receiving vaccines at the right time and using safer sex practices can prevent much mortality and morbidity. This was especially important during the COVID-19 pandemic. Research helps guide our clinical decisions and suggests an effective solution to problems.

Some viruses collaborate well with each other... but we, as humans, work together, even better.

My research with Dr. Liebenberg taught me useful research and basic sciences skills. But my research was also a valuable opportunity to reflect on medicine and life in general. Research can be fun, especially if we choose to look at our research subjects from an interesting angle (like comparing viruses to ninjas).

I have always found research to be fascinating. It requires many skills, which are fun to develop (e.g., formulating a scientific argument). Many of these skills have improved my medical writing as well. Through research, I have learned more about myself as well. I learned that I also have a love of genetics and basic sciences, in addition to clinical medicine. By asking around, I started my work in the KRISP genetics labs, one of the leading genetics labs in South Africa. Under the mentorship of Dr. Veron Ramsuran, I continued to refine my understanding of genetics and genetics research tools through a series of workshops and courses, which were incredibly fun. We extracted the DNA of a strawberry and multiplied it using a technique called polymerase chain reaction (PCR). We then repeated the process with HIV. It felt invigorating to finally apply a lab technique that we initially only knew by name. I was also exposed to many other incredible geneticists and healthcare professionals from all over the world. Through them, I learned basic coding skills, genetics ethics, and basic cloning techniques. I managed to gain all this experience, just because I took the plunge and asked if the KRISP team would take me on. I am forever grateful to work with them and to continue learning from them.

After our week in the ARV clinic, we started work in the clinics on the middle tier of the hospital complex. Some of us were allocated to the procedure room, where we helped the nurses take blood, give injections, and take blood pressure readings. My advice to any new medical student is to learn these skills as well as the language of your patients as well as you can, as soon as possible. Performing these procedures, taking patient histories, and explaining changes in treatment plans form a large part of daily clinic work.

The clinic at Northdale hospital is a dusty green waiting area (usually filled with patients) connected to a series of doctors' consultation rooms. The doctors need to push the queue and see all the patients as fast as possible. Many of the doctors and patients tend to become irritable as a result of this. The doctors just want to finish on time. The patients don't like waiting in long queues. If there is anything that I have learned from my work in the public health sector, is that patience is a virtue. Don't take the frustration of others personally. Moreover, you should never become frustrated yourself. While training with the samurai in Japan, I learned some of their important principles, which I have incorporated into my lifestyle. The word samurai originates from the word: "saburau", which means: "To serve." As medical practitioners, I believe that we serve a similar role in society, mainly by serving others. Through my reading of: "The

Art of War" and my martial arts training, I learned that controlling one's emotions is critical in any conflict situation. Getting angry and frustrated with patients or colleagues achieves nothing and shows weakness. We must strive to be level-headed and patient with all our patients and colleagues. Granted, this is not always easy. During my time in the clinic, I was asked to examine a man with epilepsy (a condition that causes people to have recurrent seizures). He visited the clinic with his mother, who was quite frustrated, after waiting in the queue for about an hour. She refused to let me see her son's blood tests because she felt that I was taking time away from her consultation (even after I reassured her that I could push her to the front of the queue). She even tried to push me away. According to the ethical principle of patient autonomy, we as healthcare providers must respect our patients' decisions. There is no point in getting frustrated. I lead the patient and his mother to the front of the queue and allowed the intern on call to help them further.

Of course, many doctors experience much more serious altercations with patients and colleagues. I was once pushed aside by a wide-eyed, half-naked psychiatry patient who fled from two security guards, at Addington hospital. For some, reason, he thought he could escape the hospital by running into the pediatric ward (which is on the 12th floor of the hospital). The security guards eventually pinned him to the ground. Some doctors call these psychiatry patients: "runners." A delirious elderly woman tried to bite me once and another claimed that he was the prophet of doom…psychiatry patients are fun. During my 4th-year pediatrics block, we needed to wash out a young girl's ear that was obstructed by a plug of earwax. She was about 6 years old, but it took at least 4 strong adults to hold her down. Never underestimate the strength of patients. Some of my friends have joked that learning martial arts should be a compulsory block in medical school. You may come across many patients who will test your patience. Remember that one of the reasons why we follow the path of a healthcare professional is to help people. When you choose not to succumb to your anger, you show others your strength of character.

Most of the patients I met in the clinic were diagnosed with chronic conditions like high blood pressure and diabetes. These are complex diseases with multifactorial causes. Managing patients with these conditions will require you to work with them a lot, over a long time, to come up with a plan for helping them (shared decision making). It takes a lot of careful coaxing and discussion to encourage a patient to stop smoking or to eat less cake to lose weight.

One of our other tasks was to find a problem in the hospital and write a report about it. We identified a patient who was given an incorrect drug dosage in the ARV clinic. Many public healthcare facilities in South Africa lack sufficient resources. You won't always have the healthcare equipment that you need. Mistakes happen in hospitals. Understandably, some doctors feel overwhelmed by the pressure of managing large numbers of patients, with only the bare minimum. It can also be seen as an opportunity to practice resourcefulness and prioritize teamwork (e.g., sharing patient caseloads fairly among colleagues). In the pediatric ward at Edendale hospital, there was only one handheld machine for checking bilirubin levels (a substance with a yellow pigment that can sometimes accumulate in tissues and cause problems). The interns needed to trust each other to monitor the battery life carefully and use the machine only when necessary. They co-operated well. Trust is important. In the obstetrics wards, the interns covered for each other, whenever one of their colleagues called in sick. The sense of camaraderie in some public hospital departments is inspiring, despite the challenges that they face.

Our final few days of the primary healthcare block were spent in the medical outpatient department. Much like most of the other departments, it was packed. On most days, it was teeming with interns in scrubs, consultants, and wave-after wave of emergency cases. It was a cacophony of beeping monitors, groaning trauma patients, and doctors and nurses calling out to each other. The energy in the air was palpable. We were given an orientation by one of the consultants. My brother and I were a few minutes late because we had some trouble finding the MOPD at first. We thought we were going to be in trouble, but we endeared ourselves to the consultant. He was Cuban and was pleasantly surprised by our ability to speak basic Spanish (another example of the importance of diversifying one's skillset). My knowledge of basic Spanish also helped me befriend another charismatic Cuban doctor, who helped manage the surgery clinics at Greys Hospital. Through him, I learnt much about the fascinating and unpredictable medical landscape in Cuba as well as life in Cuba, during the rule of Fidel Castro. He also taught me about a delicious Cuban dish which contains pork and black beans. Many Cuban students work in South African hospitals.

We started our work in MOPD by triaging the patients. We needed to assess patients for the severity of their conditions and prioritize them for treatment accordingly. People limped into the waiting room covered in blood or were carried to us in their family members' arms. There was an unconscious woman who needed to be carried to us by her spouse because there were no available wheelchairs. Another patient lost his finger in a car crash. One patient was brought to us on a stretcher after being stabbed in the chest. We needed to help decompress his lung, before the pleural space (a fluid-filled space between the lungs and the chest wall) filled with air and blood. That could have killed him. Luckily, he survived...just barely. I helped a few pregnant patients who needed to be examined with an ultrasound machine. We later discovered that they had miscarriages.

MOPD made us truly appreciate the inexhaustible vastness of medicine. You never know what condition a patient will present with. You have to be ready for anything, which is both exciting and intimidating. It is also liberating to be able to explain a patient's condition down to a molecular level. It makes you feel powerful to make the correct diagnosis and actively help a patient feel better. It is exhilarating chaos.

15

FINAL YEAR

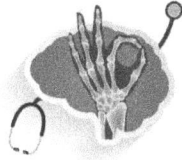

"The end is just the beginning"

— *T.S. ELIOT*

On my first day of medical school, I made sure to remember as much of that day as I could so that I could note how much I changed, by the time I reached my final year. I am not the same person I was on that fateful day back in the L7 lecture venue.

6 years of medical school is a long time. Every day was filled with new opportunities and surprises. Thousands of hours were spent studying, writing examinations, clerking patients, discussing cases, writing reports, drawing blood, consoling patients, researching, travelling, making new friends, suffering, falling in love, learning new things and so much more.

My adventures in medical school and abroad have taken me to the land of the dead, the land of the well, and the thin line that separates both of them when a person holds on to their final moments of life. During my time in medical school, I have met countless patients, healthcare workers, and other amazing people, who have fundamentally changed my views of the world and medicine. Some have helped me. Some have berated me. Others have done both. I have had the privilege of meeting some of the world's most prominent scientists through my research with CAPRISA and the KRISP labs. I explored the world of genetics. I became a TV presenter, a writer, a voice actor, a pianist, a student of Northern Long Fist Kung Fu, and many more things, to understand myself and other people better. Whenever people ask me why I wanted to study medicine, I say: "I love science and I love people." People are a central element of medicine. I believe that you have to love people if you want to love medicine and perform your best at it.

My clinical rotations exposed me to all types of people from neonates to the elderly. Each age group has unique needs that we must learn, to help them. From year 1 of medical school to year 6, I have learned basic sciences, how to become a professional as well as the medical theory necessary to effectively assess a patient clinically. There is a popular saying among doctors: "The human body doesn't change much." Granted, some things in medicine don't change much, but people change a lot. Societies change. Technology changes. Our understanding of medicine changes continuously. The onus is on us to continuously develop ourselves. Every discipline that I learned taught me something profound about medicine and life itself, which inspired my reflections in each chapter of this book.

One reason why I love medicine is because of its inexhaustible variety. There is always someone new to meet and something/someone to teach you something every day. And you can feel yourself improving when you put in the effort. In my 4th year, I drew out a protocol for clinical thinking, which helped me approach clinical questions. That was the product of years of refining my knowledge of basic and clinical sciences. I managed to publish a few articles, after having endured much trial and error, to learn the medical writing process. Medicine transforms us, but we have to invest time and effort if we want to improve. This is true, regardless of which medical school you attend. This is one of the most important lessons that I learned in medical school. I know this to be true because there have been several UKZN medical students who have also achieved great success in other prominent medical and scientific institutions abroad. They inspire me as well.

Another important lesson that I learned in medical school is that one must always ask oneself the question: "How can I use this knowledge in real life?" If one does not know the answer to something, one must also ask: "Can I find out the answer?" Medical school, like any other university, assesses your ability to learn and apply knowledge, to determine if you qualify for a degree. These systems of assessment are not always perfect. The theory is different from the practical. The real test is real life when you have to use these skills. No clinical exam (that we know of so far) can perfectly replicate the experience of resuscitating a dying patient. I recall one incident in Prince Mshiyeni hospital when I needed to apply my knowledge of basic chemistry, to see if a patient was suffering from metabolic acidosis (a condition that can cause the blood to become too acidic). If I was a doctor who did not know that information, my treatment of the patient would have been insufficient. One learns large volumes of information in medical school. With practice and experience, you will see what information is most relevant to you in your setting. Nonetheless, a certain base level of medical knowledge is expected of all healthcare professionals. This may differ between medical facilities and universities, but they will all have some commonalities. For example, every doctor should have the knowledge and skills to save a life, in an emergency. I remind myself that every day is an opportunity to apply what I have learned in medical school. Whenever a friend or family member asks you a question like: "How does high salt intake cause high blood pressure?" that is an opportunity to practice your knowledge of basic human physiology (how the human body normally works), pathophysiology (how a disease process works) as well as your communication skills. These real-life opportunities to use your knowledge help you in medical school a lot. I slowly realized that medical school and real life are very different. In medical school, there are tests and exams. You may make some mistakes. You get your results. Yes, it is incredibly important to perform well in your exams, which to some degree objectively test your medical skills and knowledge. However, this process can lull students into a false sense of security. In real life, the consequences become more serious than an exam result. A patient's life may hang in the balance. Medical school is safe and predictable. There are scheduled lectures, tutorials, and exam dates. In real life, a great responsibility is suddenly thrust upon us. There are new unpredictable situations. You may be called to the wards for a sudden emergency case. It's what we do that matters, not just our credentials or our results.

When I first enrolled in medical school, I started to wonder what life was like for medical students elsewhere in the world. Was I learning enough to be able to treat patients as well as the medical students in developed countries? One must never forget that we must use all the tools that are available to us if we wish to maximize our chances of success. The internet and social media are incredibly powerful resources that can be the cause of great suffering as well as great success. It depends on how we choose to use them. Many of my views of medicine and healthcare around the world were fundamentally changed by prominent medical writers, bloggers, and vloggers from around the world, who shared their insights into the global landscape of health. Many of them are my age and endured the same challenges that I did in medical school. By listening to their thoughts, stories, and experiences, I learned new approaches to overcoming personal challenges, such as how to manage my time better, how to use more evidence-based study strategies to improve my exam results, and how to avoid procrastination. I learned the value of using my video editing skills to create educational YouTube videos to help tutor my peers. These are just a few examples. You never know what new skills you can learn if you just take the time to listen to others, especially people who live in a different environment. By accepting knowledge from many sources, our chances of creating novel solutions to problems increase. By working together, we all become stronger.

I have only achieved what I have achieved because of the people who helped me and supported me. My family, my lecturers, my tutors, friends, consultants…the list goes on. My efforts are a product of their investment in me. In response, I do my best to help them and improve the world for others. I consider myself privileged to have received the help that I did. Many others do not receive those same opportunities. I remind myself that by improving the world for others, others will gain the opportunities to help themselves and others as well. It is an upstream solution. By helping others, we also help ourselves. Many of my closest friends in medical school came from impoverished backgrounds. Through sheer hard work and government financial support, many of them were accepted into medical school and eventually graduated. Some of them returned to their homes in rural areas, where they serve as the only doctors in their communities. Some of these villages are small, with a few scattered settlements separated by vast beautiful savannah. My friends have told me how their villages celebrate and support students who are accepted into medical school. It is because they know that one person can change a community and vice versa. Some have broken through the poverty cycle. I have seen them shed tears when they post pictures on social media of the first car that they bought (often the first car ever bought in their family). UKZN graduation ceremonies have become legendary for the unique way in which students celebrate when their names are announced and they finally hold their degrees in their hands. You need only search for the videos on YouTube to understand what I mean. At that moment, years of painstaking endeavor in the face of seemingly insurmountable odds, culminate into a glorious moment of catharsis. Students cheer, perform traditional dances in front of the entire university and even bring their parents and grandparents on stage to accept their degrees with them. Their faces glow with an overwhelming radiance. Their joy is tangible. It feels as if their bodies are suddenly infused with the combined energies of their loved ones and those who gave their all to see their children achieve greatness. It is a humbling and inspiring sight that brings tears to the eyes. It is a moving reminder that one person can change the lives of those around them.

I wrote these last few thoughts during my final year of medical school. My work continues in the hospitals and clinics of Durban.

In my final year, I revisited all of the same disciplines that I studied over the first 5 years of medical school. It felt almost like I reacquainted myself with old friends, who taught me valuable lessons about life and different people: Internal medicine, surgery, psychiatry, obstetrics, pediatrics, neonatology, primary healthcare. Returning to Durban for my final medical school clinical rotations felt cathartic.

I plan to complete two years of internship and one year of community service in South Africa. Then who knows? I intend to specialize in a field that appeals most to me. I also plan to travel abroad and learn more about medicine that is practiced overseas. That is another reason why I love medicine. There is so much potential to explore your interests while helping others.

I ask myself now: "Did I achieve all the 6 core competencies that I mentioned at the start of this book?" I would like to say that I am confident that I have developed these core competencies well, but I have a long way to go. Mastering all of them is a different question entirely. I feel that will be a lifelong pursuit, which I welcome. With each passing year, I find myself asking the question: "What is my purpose?" more often. As someone who grew up in a privileged background, I consider myself fortunate to have experienced many of the opportunities that lead me to where I am today. I believe that by healing people, developing a holistic view of health, and promoting good health in society, we give people more chances to improve our world. People will live longer and better if we do our jobs well. Mono no aware reminds us that life is impermanent. We must value every moment of it, but we must not forget to ask ourselves what will happen afterward. Seeing the world from the Chinese City of the Dead made me ponder this. Modern medicine is built on millennia of living systems that change and evolve. I am learning from the legacies of generations of pioneers who lived before me. We, too, can leave powerful and lasting legacies.

Every day, we learn something new in medicine. We are constantly building on what we know and breaking new grounds. There is no end to what we can discover. This book is just one example of how I intend to leave a legacy for future healthcare professionals. The ways we learn to heal others and master our art will change. The COVID-19 pandemic was a clear example of that. But I believe that the human experience of medicine will remain very similar. Medicine is filled with moments of great joy, like the first meeting between a mother and her newborn child. It is also filled with moments of great sorrow, like seeing death for the first time. It is also filled with every other feeling on the emotional spectrum. There are times when you will feel stressed because of an overwhelming workload or celebrate because you helped someone live longer, by giving them the right treatment. You may fall in love and enjoy the ensuing emotional rollercoaster of balancing work with your family time. You may make countless friends who study medical and non-medical disciplines and learn things you never thought existed. You may travel and learn ways of healing that aren't taught in any medical school. There will be late nights and other days when you finish early and have more than enough time to pursue your hobbies. You will experience the glamour of a well-respected profession, even if most of your time is spent covered in other people's blood. A chicken may fly into your emergency room. You'll savor that ah-ha moment when you finally understand a difficult concept, from one of your countless textbooks. You could get a big break and become one of the world's wealthiest doctors. You will have life-changing experiences if you seek them out…

Medicine brings us an infinite variety of opportunities and the hope and promises that we will meet people and learn lessons that fundamentally change our souls. But seizing those opportunities is a decision that you alone can make. Medicine is a lifelong adventure that can make us more than what we are if we choose to make it so. Learning does not end in medical school and that makes it all the more fun. We can choose to be happy at the end of a long day in the operating room. We can choose to become the best doctors we can be. We can choose to embark on one of the greatest adventures in life, which medicine can offer us.

Now that medical school is nearly done, I find it interesting that I mostly recall good memories-memories of incredible stories that I chose to make with amazing people. Any suffering that was endured just made me stronger. That is how we grow, by pushing ourselves beyond our limits-whether it be studying at our desks or investing an extra hour to examine patients when everyone else has left the wards.

When I asked myself 6 years before: "What do I want to achieve by the end of my final year?" I thought that there would be a straight path to reaching my goals. By reflecting on my experiences, I see now that the path is forever changing. It evolves with us. It arborizes like new neural connections that are constantly forming in our brains, especially as we take on new and unexpected opportunities and calculated risks. Everyone's path is different and is largely dictated by our choices. My path will vary significantly from yours. If you choose to write a book in medical school, no-one can stop you. If you want to leave a lasting legacy as a great doctor, no-one can stop you. Never let anything or anyone stop you. Medical school can be a great odyssey if you want it to be and are willing to do everything it takes to make it so.

But we must never forget that this is an odyssey that we never need to experience alone. I wrote this book to ease the journey, to leave a breadcrumb trail for those who choose to travel this path.

Like the cells that make us who we are, we are still incredibly complex as individuals, with our own unique stories, choices, and adventures. Together, we create limitless possibilities. Medicine is one life-changing way to explore ourselves-to discover those possibilities. It is an odyssey of our making.

ACKNOWLEDGMENTS

I could only write this book because of the constant support of my family, mentors, friends, teachers, and patients. Dad, Nalini, Ishq, Papa, Argie; you have always been there for me, since the beginning. I achieved all of this, because of your love and kindness.

To my mentors, Dr. Lenine Liebenberg, Dr. Veron Ramsuran and Dr. Reina Abraham, I wish to thank you for your patience and for enduring my numerous questions and emails. You both also opened my eyes to the beauty of medical writing, the world of genetics and the basic sciences as well as clinical methods.

Thank you to the African Essence team. I will be forever grateful to you all. I owe much to my teachers, who have helped me throughout my scholastic career, in school, and the wards.

I want to express my gratitude to all my medical school friends for all the busts and loyal friendship. Thank you to Mr. Gregg Davies for the amazing book jacket design and your hard work.

Last, but certainly not least, I thank the countless patients who have taught me so much. You continue to galvanize my spirit and inspire countless medical students to change the world.

SOURCES

1. HOW IT ALL STARTED

- Kavic MS. Competency and the six core competencies. *JSLS*. 2002;6(2):95–97.

2. INTERPERSONAL AND COMMUNICATION SKILLS

- Ziegelstein RC. Creating Structured Opportunities for Social Engagement to Promote Well-Being and Avoid Burnout in Medical Students and Residents. Academic medicine: journal of the Association of American Medical Colleges. 2018;93(4):537-9.
- Choudhary A, Gupta V. Teaching communications skills to medical students: Introducing the fine art of medical practice. *Int J Appl Basic Med Res*. 2015;5(Suppl 1): S41–S44. doi:10.4103/2229-516X.162273
- Dyche L. Interpersonal skill in medicine: the essential partner of verbal communication. *J Gen Intern Med*.

2007;22(7):1035–1039. doi:10.1007/s11606-007-0153-0

3. BALANCE

- Cisneros V, Goldberg I, Schafenacker A, Bota RG. Balancing Life and Medical School. *Mental Illness*. 2015;7(1):5768. doi:10.4081/mi.2015.5768

4. THE PRECLINICAL YEARS

- Kavic MS. Competency and the six core competencies. JSLS. 2002;6(2):95–97.

5. PEDIATRICS

- Health K-NDo. History of Addington hospital 2001 [Available from: http://www.kznhealth.gov.za/Addington/history.htm.

6. GYNAECOLOGY

- Torday JS. On the evolution of development. *Trends Dev Biol*. 2014;8:17-37.

7. ACUTE INTEGRATED HEALTH

- Pallett PM, Link S, Lee K. New "golden" ratios for facial beauty. *Vision Res*. 2010;50(2):149-154. doi:10.1016/j.visres.2009.11.003
- Seshadri KG. The neuroendocrinology of love. *Indian J*

Endocrinol Metab. 2016;20(4):558-563. doi:10.4103/2230-8210.183479

- de Boer A, van Buel EM, Ter Horst GJ. Love is more than just a kiss: a neurobiological perspective on love and affection. *Neuroscience.* 2012;201:114-124. doi:10.1016/j.neuroscience.2011.11.017
- Maestripieri D. The Evolutionary History of Love 2012. Available from: https://www.psychologytoday. com/za/blog/games-primates-play/201203/the-evolutionary-history-love?amp.
- Langeslag, Sandra & Van Strien, Jan. (2016). Regulation of Romantic Love Feelings: Preconceptions, Strategies, and Feasibility. PLOS ONE. 11. e0161087. 10.1371/journal.pone.0161087.

8. PRIMARY HEALTH CARE

- World Health Organization. Primary Health Care 2019 [Available from: https://www.who.int/news-room/fact-sheets/detail/primary-health-care.
- *Reygaert WC. An overview of the antimicrobial resistance mechanisms of bacteria. AIMS microbiology. 2018;4(3):482-501.*
- *Hill MR, Goicochea S, Merlo LJ. In their own words: stressors facing medical students in the millennial generation. Med Educ Online. 2018;23(1):1530558. doi:10.1080/10872981.2018.1530558*
- *TBFACTS.ORG. TB Statistics South Africa - National, incidence, provincial 2020 [Available from: https://tbfacts.org/tb-statistics-south-africa/.*
- The Discovery of PCR: ProCuRement of Divine Power. *Dig Dis Sci.* 2015;60(8):2230-1.
- Mendoza-Gallegos RA, Rios A, Garcia-Cordero JL. An Affordable and Portable Thermocycler for Real-Time

PCR Made of 3D-Printed Parts and Off-the-Shelf Electronics. Analytical Chemistry. 2018;90(9):5563-8.

- Rampersad J, Wang X, Gayadeen H, Ramsewak S, Ammons D. In-house polymerase chain reaction for affordable and sustainable Chlamydia trachomatis detection in Trinidad and Tobago. Revista panamericana de salud publica = Pan American journal of public health. 2007;22(5):317-22.
- Kalis B, Collier M, Fu R. 10 Promising AI Applications in Health Care: Harvard Business Review; 2018 [Available from: https://hbr.org/2018/05/10-promising-ai-applications-in-health-care.]

9. INTERNAL MEDICINE

- Cartwright M. Ninja 2019 [Accessed 9 April, 2020]. Available from: https://www.ancient.eu/Ninja/.
- Grabianowski E. How Ninja work [Accessed 10 April, 2020]. Available from: https://people.howstuffworks.com/ninja.htm.
- Sun-Tzu, Griffith, S. B. The Art of War. Oxford, Clarendon Press; 1964.

10. SURGERY

- Mousavizadeh L, Ghasemi S. Genotype and phenotype of COVID-19: Their roles in pathogenesis [published online ahead of print, 2020 Mar 31]. *J Microbiol Immunol Infect.* 2020;S1684-1182(20)30082-7.
- Frieman M. The art of war: battles between virus and host. *Curr Opin Virol.* 2014;6:76–77. doi:10.1016/j.coviro.2014.05.001
- Dela Cruz CS. The Art of War on Viruses. Science

Translational Medicine. 2014; 6(244): 244ec118-244ec118. doi:10.1016/j.jmii.2020.03.022

- Cleemput S, Dumon W, Fonseca V, et al. Genome Detective Coronavirus Typing Tool for rapid identification and characterization of novel coronavirus genomes. Bioinformatics (Oxford, England). 2020.
- Epstein, D. J. (2019). *Range: Why generalists triumph in a specialized world.*
- Patient-centered medicine. A professional evolution.*Laine C, Davidoff F JAMA. 1996 Jan 10; 275(2):152-6.*
- Buetow S, Elwyn G. The window-mirror: a new model of the patient-physician relationship. *Open Med.* 2008;2(1):e20-e25.
- Beauchamp TL, Childress JF. Principles of biomedical ethics.Oxford: Oxford University Press; 2001
- Jonsen A, Toulmin S. The abuse of casuistry: a history of moral reasoning. Berkeley: University of California Press; 1988.
- Rawls J. The law of peoples; with, the idea of public reason revisited. Cambridge (MA): Harvard University Press; 1999.
- Personal illness narratives: using reflective writing to teach empathy .*DasGupta S, Charon R. Acad Med. 2004 Apr; 79(4):351-6.*
- Personal growth in medical faculty: a qualitative study. *Kern DE, Wright SM, Carrese JA, Lipkin M Jr, Simmons JM, Novack DH, Kalet A, Frankel R West J Med. 2001 Aug; 175(2):92-8.*
- Decety J, Fotopoulou A. Why empathy has a beneficial impact on others in medicine: unifying theories. *Front Behav Neurosci.* 2015;8:457. Published 2015 Jan 14. doi:10.3389/fnbeh.2014.00457
- Beckes L., Coan J. A. (2011). Social baseline theory: the role of social proximity in emotion and economy of

action. Soc. Personal. Psychol. Compass 5, 976–988
10.1111/j.1751-9004.2011.00400.x

- Coan J. A. (2011). "The social regulation of emotion,"
  in The Oxford Handbook of Social Neuroscience, eds
  Decety J., Cacioppo J. T. (New York: Oxford University
  Press;), 614–623
- The neurobiology of stress and development. *Gunnar
  M, Quevedo KAnnu Rev Psychol. 2007; 58():145-73.*
- Influence of social support and emotional context on
  pain processing and magnetic brain responses in
  fibromyalgia.*Montoya P, Larbig W, Braun C, Preissl H,
  Birbaumer NArthritis Rheum. 2004 Dec; 50(12):4035-44.*
- A picture's worth: partner photographs reduce
  experimentally induced pain.*Master SL,Eisenberger NI,
  Taylor SE, Naliboff BD, Shirinyan D, Lieberman MDPsychol
  Sci. 2009 Nov; 20(11):1316-8.*
- Viewing pictures of a romantic partner reduces
  experimental pain: involvement of neural reward
  systems. *Younger J, Aron A, Parke S, Chatterjee N, Mackey
  SPLoS One. 2010 Oct 13; 5(10):e13309.*
- The free-energy principle: a unified brain theory?*Friston
  KNat Rev Neurosci. 2010 Feb; 11(2):127-38.*

11. PSYCHIATRY

- John Cookson,1 - A brief history of psychiatry,
  Editor(s): Pádraig Wright, Julian Stern, Michael
  Phelan,Core Psychiatry (Third Edition),W.B.
  Saunders,2012,Pages 3-11,ISBN
  9780702033971,https://doi.org/10.1016/B978-0-
  7020-3397-1.00001X.(http://www.sciencedirect.com/
  science/article/pii/B978070203397100001X)
- Groopman J. The Troubled History of Psychiatry: The
  New Yorker; 2019.

- Shorter E. History of psychiatry. *Curr Opin Psychiatry.* 2008;21(6):593-597. doi:10.1097/YCO.0b013e32830aba12
- Pacheco JP, Giacomin HT, Tam WW, et al. Mental health problems among medical students in Brazil: a systematic review and meta-analysis. *Braz J Psychiatry.* 2017;39(4):369-378. doi:10.1590/1516-4446-2017-2223
- Health-related quality of life of students from a private medical school in Brazil.*Lins L, Carvalho FM, Menezes MS, Porto-Silva L, Damasceno H Int J Med Educ. 2015 Nov 8; 6():149-54.*
- Tempski P, Bellodi PL, Paro HB, Enns SC, Martins MA, Schraiber LB. What do medical students think about their quality of life? A qualitative study. BMC Med Educ. 2012;12:106–106.

12. NEONATOLOGY

- Palmer B, Quinn Griffin MT, Reed P, Fitzpatrick JJ. Self-transcendence and work engagement in acute care staff registered nurses. Crit Care Nurs Q. 2010 Apr-Jun;33(2):138-47. doi: 10.1097/CNQ.0b013e3181d912d8. PMID: 20234203.

13. OBSTETRICS

- Cohen B, Seibel MM. A Historical Perspective of Obstetrics and Gynecology: A Backdrop for Reproductive Technology. In: Seibel MM, Bernstein J, editors. Technology and Infertility: Clinical, Psychosocial, Legal, and Ethical Aspects. New York, NY: Springer New York; 1993. p. 1-9

14. COMMUNITY HEALTH

- Griffiths DJ. Endogenous retroviruses in the human genome sequence. Genome Biol. 2001;2(6):REVIEWS1017. doi:10.1186/gb-2001-2-6-reviews1017
- Mi S, Lee X, Li X, Veldman GM, Finnerty H, Racie L, LaVallie E, Tang XY, Edouard P, Howes S, et al. Syncytin is a captive retroviral envelope protein involved in human placental morphogenesis. Nature. 2000;403:785–789. doi: 10.1038/35001608.
- de Oliveira, T. et al. Transmission networks and risk of HIV infection in KwaZulu-Natal, South Africa: a community-wide phylogenetic study. Lancet HIV 4, e41–e50 (2017).
- UN Joint Programme on HIV/AIDS (UNAIDS). Ending AIDS: Progress Towards the 90–90–90 Targets. (2017).
- Shisana, O. et al. South African National HIV Prevalence, Incidence and Behaviour Survey, 2012. (HSRC Press, 2014).
- Lackner AA, Lederman MM, Rodriguez B. HIV pathogenesis: the host. *Cold Spring Harb Perspect Med*. 2012;2(9):a007005. Published 2012 Sep 1. doi:10.1101/cshperspect.a007005
- Bruni, L. et al. Human papillomavirus and related diseases in the world. Summ. Rep. 27(July), 2017
- Zur Hausen, H. Papillomaviruses in the causation of human cancers—a brief historical account. Virology 384, 260–265 (2009).
- Hebner CM, Laimins LA. Human papillomaviruses: basic mechanisms of pathogenesis and oncogenicity. Reviews in medical virology. 2006;16(2):83-97.

- Clifford, G., Franceschi, S., Diaz, M., Muñoz, N. & Villa, L. L. Chapter 3: HPV type-distribution in women with and without cervical neoplastic diseases. Vaccine 24, S26–S34 (2006).
- Liebenberg, Lenine & McKinnon, Lyle & Yende-Zuma, Nonhlanhla & Garrett, Nigel & Baxter, Cheryl & Kharsany, Ayesha & Archary, Moherndran & Rositch, Anne & Samsunder, Natasha & Mansoor, Leila & Passmore, Jo-Ann & Abdool Karim, Salim & Abdool Karim, Quarraisha. (2019). HPV infection and the genital cytokine milieu in women at high risk of HIV acquisition. Nature Communications. 10. 10.1038/s41467-019-13089-2.

15. FINAL YEAR

- Evans HM. Wonder and the clinical encounter. *Theor Med Bioeth*. 2012;33(2):123-136. doi:10.1007/s11017-012-9214-4